Sue Righthand, PhD
Bruce Kerr, PhD
Kerry Drach, PsyD

Child Maltreatment Risk Assessments
An Evaluation Guide

Pre-publication
REVIEWS,
COMMENTARIES,
EVALUATIONS . . .

"**T**he value of this guide lies in the wealth of conceptual, empirical, and practical information that the authors present in a clear and concise manner. The material is current and represents state-of-the-art theory and practice. The authors appropriately pay considerable attention to the distinction between legal and clinical risks assessments, and present numerous 'cautionary notes' related to the practice of risk assessment. The material in this book goes far beyond child maltreatment risk assessment, including material on the impact of child maltreatment, spouse abuse, and the effectiveness of interventions.

Chapter 5, which provides many guidelines, forms, and practical tips related to risk assessment, will be especially valuable to risk assessment professionals. I recommend this guide as a must-read instructional text for individuals who desire to learn about child maltreatment clinical risk assessment. This book also will be an important resource (and reminder of salient risk assessment issues) for seasoned professionals who are currently engaging in child maltreatment risk assessment."

Joel S. Milner, PhD
Professor of Psychology;
Distinguished Research Professor;
Director, Center for the Study of Family
Violence and Sexual Assault,
Northern Illinois University

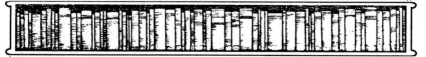

More pre-publication
REVIEWS, COMMENTARIES, EVALUATIONS . . .

"**T**his book is essential reading for clinicians and forensic examiners who see cases involving issues related to child maltreatment. The authors have compiled an impressive critical survey of the relevant research on child maltreatment. Their material is well organized into sections on definitions, impact, risk assessment, and risk management. Their combined clinical wisdom is evident in the final chapter, titled 'Putting It All Together.' This book represents a giant step toward promoting evidence-based evaluation, treatment, and testimony."

Diane H. Schetky, MD
Professor of Psychiatry,
University of Vermont College of Medicine;
Private Practice, Forensic Psychiatry

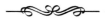

"**T**his is a successfully ambitious, comprehensive book that distills a vast amount of clinical research and experience into a focused and pragmatic guide to conducting child maltreatment risk assessments. The authors describe and weave together 'best practices' in areas including violence risk assessment, forensic evalua-

tion, and clinical intervention to provide a thoughtful and sophisticated framework for conducting these often complex, high-stakes assessments. The final chapter is a much-needed road map for conducting child maltreatment risk assessments that also includes a frank discussion of the controversies and pitfalls that can complicate professional practice in this specialized assessment area. This book will be invaluable to clinicians who conduct child maltreatment risk assessments, professionals who supervise or teach others how to conduct these assessments, and attorneys and judges who must rely upon these assessments when making far-reaching decisions about the lives of children and families."

Robert Kinscherff, PhD, JD
Director of Juvenile Court
Clinic Services, Juvenile Court
Department, Massachusetts Trial Court;
Director, Forensic Specialization
Program, Massachusetts School
of Professional Psychology; Lecturer,
Boston University School of Law;
Clinical Associate in Psychology,
Harvard Medical School

HMTP

The Haworth Maltreatment and Trauma Press®
An Imprint of The Haworth Press, Inc.
New York • London • Oxford

Child Maltreatment Risk Assessments
An Evaluation Guide

Child Maltreatment Risk Assessments
An Evaluation Guide

Sue Righthand, PhD
Bruce Kerr, PhD
Kerry Drach, PsyD

HMTP

The Haworth Maltreatment and Trauma Press®
An Imprint of The Haworth Press, Inc.
New York • London • Oxford

Published by

The Haworth Maltreatment and Trauma Press®, an imprint of The Haworth Press, Inc., 10 Alice Street, Binghamton, NY 13904-1580.

Cover design by Jennifer M. Gaska.

Library of Congress Cataloging-in-Publication Data

Righthand, Sue.
    Child maltreatment risk assessments : an evaluation guide / Sue Righthand, Bruce Kerr, Kerry Drach.
        p. cm.
    Includes bibliographical references and index.
    ISBN 0-7890-1215-4 (hard : alk. paper)—ISBN 0-7890-1216-2 (soft : alk. paper)
    1. Child abuse—Prevention. 2. Child abuse—Investigation. 3. Abused children—Health risk assessment. 4. Family assessment. 5. Abusive parents—Behavior modification. 6. Abused children—Rehabilitation. I. Kerr, Bruce, 1952- II. Drach, Kerry. III. Title.

HV6626.5 .R54 2003
362.76'5—dc21
                                                                        2002027642

CONTENTS

Preface

Child Maltreatment Risk Assessments: An Evaluation Guide is a professional practice manual designed to assist in forensic risk assessment in child maltreatment cases. The book is divided into an introduction and five chapters. The Introduction discusses procedural issues in the field of child maltreatment. Chapter 1 defines the concept of child maltreatment. Chapter 2 discusses the impact child maltreatment may have on children and their development. Chapter 3 reviews the empirical literature on risk factors associated with child maltreatment. Chapter 4 discusses the research pertaining to treatment possibilities and risk management strategies. Chapter 5 provides an introduction to forensic assessments and highlights issues important for conducting and writing high-quality, ethical evaluations in child maltreatment cases.

This book was written to provide a convenient, empirically based evaluation guide. The approach has been, wherever possible, to draw upon the research literature in this area and direct practicing clinicians and students toward that literature. Thus, the goal of this book is to provide practicing clinicians and students with a convenient and up-to-date review of the literature and discussion of the pragmatics of professional work in this area. This book also will serve readers as a continuing reference source for work in this area.

ABOUT THE AUTHORS

Sue Righthand, PhD, is a licensed clinical psychologist in private practice in Rockland, Maine, and holds an adjunct faculty position in the University of Maine's Department of Psychology. Dr. Righthand has extensive experience evaluating children and parents in forensic settings and serves as a consultant to the Maine District Court's Family Division, working with the court to develop a system to facilitate timely, high quality forensic assessments in child welfare cases. She directs a needs and risk assessment project pertaining to Maine juveniles who have sexually offended.

Dr. Righthand received the United States Department of Health and Human Services Commissioner's Award in 1996 for outstanding leadership and service in the prevention of child abuse and neglect and the Maine Child Abuse Action Network Professional of the Year Award in 2000. She is co-author of *Juveniles Who Have Sexually Offended: A Review of the Professional Literature* and the *Juvenile Sex Offender Assessment Protocol.*

Bruce B. Kerr, PhD, is a licensed clinical psychologist in private practice in Kennebunk, Maine. He performs child maltreatment, child homicide, and other forensic evaluations for the Maine State and Federal Courts. Dr. Kerr has served two terms on the Maine Family Law Advisory Commission and has provided continuing education to mental health and legal professionals on a range of subjects related to forensic psychology.

Kerry M. Drach, PsyD, has worked in the field of child abuse assessment and treatment since 1977. He is senior psychologist with the Spurwink Child Abuse Program in Portland, Maine, a multidisciplinary forensic child abuse evaluation program, and has extensive experience evaluating children and parents in the context of child maltreatment proceedings. Dr. Drach's research interests include the role of sexual behavior problems in sexual abuse diagnosis, and psychosocial and psychometric characteristics of maltreating parents.

Acknowledgments

Preparation of this document was supported, in part, by a federal child abuse and neglect grant from the Office of Child Abuse and Neglect in the Children's Bureau of the U.S. Department of Health and Human Services Administration for Children and Families and through the administrative support of the Maine Department of Human Services and the Maine State Forensic Service.

The authors would like to especially acknowledge and thank Sandra Hodge, director of Child Welfare in Maine. It was because of her vision and dedication to the safety and welfare of children that this work was possible. Our special thanks also to our editor Robert Geffner for his support and recognition of the value of this work.

In addition, the authors appreciate the contributions of consultants to the State Forensic Service's Child Abuse and Neglect Evaluation Project, James Jacobs, Karen Mosher, Gary Rasmussen, and Carlann Welch for their comments and ideas on earlier versions of this book. This appreciation extends to Jeffrey Hecker who, although not a formal consultant to the project, took the time to review and comment on an early draft of this work.

We also would like to thank Debra Frace for her assistance with early drafts of this document and Mary Teleha, who provided valuable assistance through her excellent attention to detail during the proofreading process. In addition, we extend our appreciation to Pamela Richards, who was instrumental in the final stages of preparing this manuscript.

Introduction

In its most recent survey addressing the problem of child maltreatment, the *Third National Incidence Study of Child Abuse and Neglect* [NIS-3], the United States Department of Health and Human Services estimated that over 1.5 million children were abused or neglected in the United States during 1993 (Sedlack and Broadhurst, 1996). This statistic translates into 23.1 children per 1,000. In addition, the NIS-3 study estimated that, during the year under study, 1,500 children died because of child abuse or neglect.

As staggering as these figures may seem, they only represent cases known to child protective agencies or selected community professionals. These figures do not include incidences of child maltreatment that have not been reported to the child protective agencies or the categories of professionals included in the study. In addition, they do not include abusive or neglectful behaviors that have not been identified as such, either by the individuals involved or others who are aware of the behaviors.

As child maltreatment has become recognized as a major social problem, states have enacted laws providing for state intervention in cases of child abuse and neglect. Legal interventions attempt to balance child safety with the parents' rights to privacy. However, as Melton and his colleagues (1997) observed, instability and inadequacies in the foster care systems throughout the country have raised serious concerns about the efficacy of these interventions and whether they do more harm than good.

Because of the widespread concerns about children remaining in foster care for long periods of time, frequently moving from one home to the next, the United States enacted the Adoption and Safe Families Act of 1997 (ASFA) (Public Law 105-89). The ASFA set forth federal requirements to be implemented through state statutes and agency policies and procedures.

The objectives of ASFA were to address the problem of children remaining in foster care for years by reforming the child welfare system to focus directly on children's safety, permanency, and well-being

(American Bar Association, 1998). While continuing to require that states make reasonable efforts to preserve or reunify families, ASFA requirements specify that child health and safety are paramount concerns. Thus, and as exemplified in the Maine statute (Child and Family Services and Child Protection Act, 1998), the parents' right to "family integrity is limited by the right of children to be protected from abuse and neglect" (CFSCPA, 1998, p. 3).

When out-of-home placements are required, to facilitate timely, safe, and permanent child placements, ASFA enables states to cease family reunification efforts when certain aggravating circumstances, as defined by state law, are present. ASFA also permits child protection agencies to engage in concurrent planning for alternative placements that will provide the child with a safe and permanent home if family reunification is no longer an option. It further requires that reunification efforts and legal proceedings be accomplished within shortened time frames in order to reduce the time that children spend in temporary situations. How states implement ASFA may vary. It is therefore essential that professionals working with children and adults in child maltreatment cases know the relevant laws and procedures in their state.

Typically, legal proceedings in civil child maltreatment cases begin with requests for preliminary protection orders. This action requires that the court hear evidence alleging that parental action or inaction has caused or presents an immediate risk of serious injuries or harm to a child. Following the hearing, the court makes a finding as to whether a child is at immediate risk of serious abuse or neglect. If the court finds the child is at risk, it reviews proposed dispositions that may alleviate the risk, and orders those most likely to promote and ensure the child's safety and welfare.

When the risk to the child does not appear sufficient to warrant removal, the parents retain custody. Service plans are designed to address the underlying causes of parental abuse and neglect and reduce or eliminate the risk of harm to the children. If the court finds the risk to the child to be sufficient to warrant removing the child from parental custody, appropriate state agencies are responsible for developing rehabilitation, reunification, and permanency plans.

If reunification efforts are unsuccessful, or are deemed inappropriate due to the nature of the maltreatment or the needs of the child, proceedings to terminate parental rights may ensue. For example, in

Maine, state law requires the Department of Human Services to petition for termination of parental rights at the earliest time such action is indicated. The Maine statute (Child and Family Services and Child Protection Act, 1998) lists a variety of factors that indicate termination of parental rights proceedings are in order. These circumstances range from abandonment or the parent's commission of a heinous act to the court's finding that the parent is unwilling or unable to take responsibility for the child within a time frame that is reasonably sufficient to meet the child's needs.

When child maltreatment has occurred, judges, attorneys, state agencies, and parents may seek clinical evaluations to assist with the tasks of developing treatment plans and risk management strategies or making difficult decisions about termination of parental rights. Clinical child maltreatment evaluations may be requested at most any stage in the legal process and can provide empirically based findings and specialized knowledge that may assist the involved parties in arriving at decisions designed to best meet the needs of individual children and their families. Evaluations that are fair, impartial, and grounded in knowledge rather than opinion are required. The professional's challenge is to meet this need.

Child maltreatment risk assessments, as described in this guide, pertain to cases of documented child maltreatment. The procedures for forensic child maltreatment clinical evaluations described herein should not be confused with forensic investigative assessments. In the latter case, assessments typically are conducted by child protective caseworkers, law enforcement officers, and, sometimes, clinicians in order to determine whether a child has been maltreated. If the child has been maltreated, investigative assessments also attempt to ascertain the nature and circumstances of the maltreatment as well as the identity of the perpetrator or perpetrators.

In child maltreatment risk assessments referral questions typically involve an evaluation of factors that may increase or decrease the risk of continued maltreatment. In addition, recommendations for interventions that are designed to promote the child's safety and healthy development and reduce the risk of further negative outcomes are required. This guide provides a distillation of the professional literature to facilitate the work of evaluators and other professionals engaged in this work.

A word of caution is required. As Ammerman (1998) observed, "At the outset, research in the behavioral and social sciences is fraught with methodological and measurement problems" (p. 130), and difficulties conducting rigorous, well-controlled research in the area of child abuse and neglect abound. Methodological problems include an absence of consensus on clear definitions of varying types of child maltreatment. Different types of maltreatment often are combined in research studies, precluding an assessment of each one's unique effects and influences, while other confounding factors such as poverty or child and parent characteristics not directly related to the maltreatment are not controlled. Other problems include small sample sizes and samples of convenience, raising questions about whether findings from such studies can be generalized to other populations. Studies in other relevant areas, such as substance abuse and psychiatric disorders, frequently focus only on males (Azar et al., 1998), when females frequently are the focus of child maltreatment assessments. Additional methodological limitations such as infrequent randomized and longitudinal designs also may affect the reliability and validity of research findings and consequently limit our understanding of the etiology and prevention of child maltreatment.

Most of the studies presented in this guide are consistent with previous independent research. When findings are supported and replicated, confidence is increased. As Mullen and colleagues have noted (1996), "Methodologically ideal studies in this area may always escape us, but good enough studies will, when taken together, illuminate the central theoretical and clinical issues" (p. 17).

In spite of the methodological difficulties previously described, the professional literature reveals significant gains in our understanding of the factors associated with child maltreatment and, concomitantly, our ability to effectively intervene. This guide is an attempt to present this literature, with the appropriate cautions in mind, in an organized fashion in order to facilitate quality forensic evaluations in child maltreatment cases. In this way we may assist the courts and the child welfare system to advance the safety and well-being of children and their families. As Kuehnle (1998) wrote regarding child sexual abuse:

> . . . There is no single test, marker, or mathematical equation for determining whether a child has experienced . . . abuse [or for determining that a person has maltreated a child or will in the

future]. . . . The empirical data, historical information, test results, and children's [and adults'] statements must all be evaluated against a complex matrix of interrelated factors. The forensic psychologist has the responsibility to educate the court regarding the complexity of these evaluations so that the trier of fact may be assisted in rendering the ultimate decision. (p. 18)

The authors hope that this guide will help our colleagues, as well as ourselves, to achieve that goal.

Chapter 1

Child Maltreatment: What Is It?

State and federal jurisdictions have enacted laws that permit legal interventions to protect children who have been abused or neglected. However, philosophical differences among lawmakers and an absence of conceptual clarity among mental health professionals about the definitions of child abuse and neglect have resulted in vague and divergent definitions and legal standards (Melton et al., 1987, 1997). In fact, there is no consensus, professional or otherwise, about what is acceptable or adequate parenting (Azar et al., 1995; Melton et al., 1987, 1997).

Attempts to establish uniform definitions of abuse and neglect are further complicated by cultural, moral, ethnic, and class differences. For example, debates (Melton et al., 1987, 1997) about the use of corporal punishment complicate attempts to establish a definition of physical abuse. Efforts to define neglectful parenting and psychological abuse have been especially controversial, with much disagreement about what constitutes satisfactory parental behavior (Melton et al., 1987, 1997). In the absence of accepted, standardized definitions of child maltreatment, mental health professionals may be influenced by their personal conceptions of adequate parenting and ignore the cultural meanings of certain behaviors and the effects of less than optimal environmental conditions (Azar et al., 1995; Garbarino, 1997; Miller-Perrin and Perrin, 1999).

The legal basis for state intervention into parental custody and care of children, however, is risk of harm. Thus, Tymchuk (1992) has noted that in the area of abuse and neglect, parental adequacy is defined as the nonoccurrence of abuse or neglect and the occurrence of adequate health care and safety. Terms such as "minimally adequate" and "minimal parenting competence" that more accurately reflect the legal issue in question have begun to replace the more general term of "parental capacity" in the mental health profession's vocabulary

(Azar et al., 1995; Budd and Holdsworth, 1996). All of these terms, however, still lack established meaning or clear scientific basis.

In order to adequately assess the risks and needs of the families and individuals for whom child maltreatment is a problem, the behaviors in question need clear, standardized definitions. In addition, standardized terms and operational definitions are a necessary condition for research purposes so that comparative analyses can be conducted both within and across disciplines. Clear terms and definitions enable us to test our hypotheses, improve our knowledge base, enhance the accuracy of our assessments, and increase the effectiveness of our interventions.

Geffner (1996) observed that, although the study of family violence is relatively new, the broader study of human aggression and violence is much more established and clearly defined. He encouraged people working in the area of intrafamilial abuse and violence to use this existing knowledge and research base more often. Geffner also provided a suggestion to enhance conceptual clarity and uniform definitions: "Perhaps it would be better to change the term 'abuse' to 'maltreatment' to describe the acts of aggression, abuse, and trauma inflicted by one family or relationship member toward another who has less power or authority" (p. 3). He observed that this definition of family maltreatment could encompass child maltreatment as well as spouse, partner, and elder maltreatment.

Consistent with Geffner's proposal, acts of child physical abuse, sexual abuse, psychological abuse, and neglect are defined in this document as child maltreatment. Unfortunately, even this term is hampered by the lack of consensus regarding the underlying definitions of physical abuse, sexual abuse, neglect, and psychological abuse.

DEFINITIONS OF ABUSE

In their review of the historical, cultural, political, theoretical, and social scientific approaches to defining child maltreatment, Barnett and colleagues (1994) developed research definitions and severity ratings for six subtypes of child maltreatment. These subtypes included: (1) physical abuse, (2) sexual abuse, (3) failure to provide (physical neglect), (4) lack of supervision (physical neglect), (5) emotional maltreatment, and (6) moral, legal, and educational maltreatment.

Severity ratings ranged from level one, the least severe, to level five, the most severe. Examples of level one physical abuse included minor marks on a child's body, inflicted by hand or object, in the absence of marks to the child's neck or head. Level two included numerous or nonminor marks to the child's body. Level three included marks inflicted on the child's head, face, or neck, minor burns, serious bruises, minor lacerations, and parental handprints as a result of grabbing. Level four included hitting with an object likely to result in serious injury, nonminor lacerations, fractures, concussions, second degree burns, attempts to choke or smother that did not result in hospitalization, and injuries requiring hospitalization for less than twenty-four hours. Level five included injuries that necessitated hospitalization, resulted in permanent physical damage or disfigurement, or were fatal. Severity ratings for the other forms of child maltreatment were established as well.

Barnett and colleagues (1994) stressed that the objective of their work was to develop operational definitions and severity ratings of child maltreatment for research purposes, emphasizing that the terms and ratings were not intended for making clinical or legal decisions regarding whether a particular act constituted maltreatment. They also stated that they did not endorse the application of the definitions and ratings for nonresearch purposes. Thus, although these definitions are conceptually useful, they fall short of an accepted system of professional classification for use in clinical assessments, and there currently is no such system available.

The need for clear definitions of terms extends beyond research purposes. Clinical assessments of child maltreatment also require that definitions of child maltreatment be operationalized. Although child maltreatment and specific acts of child abuse and neglect are sociolegal terms, clinicians must be able to identify and articulate those parental behaviors that are highly likely to cause trauma to children and, as a consequence, warrant intervention. In response to this need, the following operational definitions of physical abuse, sexual abuse, psychological abuse, and neglect are offered to assist clinicians assessing children and parents who are affected by or have perpetrated child maltreatment. These definitions are based on a review of Barnett and colleagues' work, the U.S. Department of Health and

Human Services' *Third National Incidence Study of Child Abuse and Neglect* (NIS-3) (Sedlack and Broadhurst, 1996), and other relevant articles (e.g., Hart, Brassard, and Karlson, 1996; Hart, Brassard, Binggeli et al., 2002).

Physical Abuse

The NIS-3 (Sedlack and Broadhurst, 1996) defined physical abuse as involving acts that result in demonstrable harm or, when combined with other abusive and neglectful acts, create a moderate risk of demonstrable harm to the child. Acts were defined as including ". . . hitting with a hand, stick, strap, or other object; punching; kicking; shaking; throwing; burning; stabbing; or choking a child" (p. 2-10). The NIS-3 definition of *physical abuse* will be accepted for the purposes of this handbook.

Sexual Abuse

The NIS-3 defined sexual abuse as including three different forms of abusive behaviors: intrusion, genital molestation, and other or un-specified acts of sexual abuse. Intrusion included "oral, anal, or geni-tal penile, digital or other types of penetration" (p. 2-10). In contrast, genital molestation involved some form of genital contact, but with-out apparent penetration. The "other or unknown" sexual abuse cate-gory included acts that did not involve genital contact, such as fondling the breasts or buttocks, genital exposure, and other unspeci-fied sexual acts not thought to have involved genital contact.

The NIS-3 (Sedlack and Broadhurst, 1996) definition of sexual abuse also included inadequate or inappropriate supervision of a child's "voluntary sexual activities" in the residual sexual abuse cate-gory (p. 2-14). The present authors, however, respectfully disagree with this classification. This disagreement is based on the hypothesis that inadequate or inappropriate supervision of a child that resulted in sexual activity, or even sexual abuse, is better classified as neglect rather than sexual abuse because the behavior of the person not ade-quately supervising the child apparently lacked sexual intent.

For the purposes of this guide, only sexually abusive acts or behav-iors perpetrated by the parent or caregiver are defined as *sexual abuse*. In addition to the types of sexually abusive behaviors de-scribed above, such acts may include voyeurism, child pornography, and child prostitution. Inadequate or inappropriate supervision, such as leaving a child with sexually abusive "caregivers" or individuals, is considered here to be physical neglect.

Psychological Abuse

In addition to physical and sexual abuse, the NIS-3 (Sedlack and Broadhurst, 1996) identified one other category of abusive behavior, emotional abuse. The NIS-3 defined emotional abuse as involving three classifications. The first included close confinement, exemplified by severe forms of punishment such as tying or binding a child's arms or legs together to a piece of furniture or other object or confining a child to an enclosed area such as a closet or a basement. The second involved verbal and emotional assaults including persistent patterns of belittling, denigrating, scapegoating, and other nonphysical, but clearly hostile or rejecting, behaviors such as repeated threats of beatings, sexual assault, and abandonment. The third, residual, category included other forms of emotional abuse such as attempted sexual or physical assaults; throwing something at a child but missing; withholding shelter, sleep, or other necessities as punishment; and economic exploitation.

Hart, Brassard, and Karlson (1996) and Hart, Brassard, Binggeli et al. (2002) identified and described six categories of psychological maltreatment based upon research and professional opinions. These included the following:

1. *Spurning,* described as hostile, degrading, and rejecting behavior by a caregiver such as belittling, ridiculing, shaming, and publicly humiliating the child
2. *Terrorizing,* described as threats to physically hurt, kill, or abandon the child, exposing the child or the child's love objects to violence, or leaving a child unattended in threatening situations
3. *Exploiting or corrupting,* described as actions by the caregiver that encourage deviant behaviors such as antisocial, criminal, and self-destructive acts, promoting developmentally inappropriate behaviors such as parentifying or infantalizing the child, and interfering with or restricting developmental autonomy through extreme overinvolvement, intrusiveness, or dominance

4. *Denying emotional responsiveness,* described as ignoring a child's attempts and need to interact, interacting with the child only when absolutely essential, and behaving in a manner that is devoid of love and affection
5. *Isolating,* described as consistently placing unreasonable limits or restrictions on a child's social interactions and interfering with the child's need for peer and adult relationships
6. *Mental heath, medical, and educational neglect,* described as refusing, failing to seek, or ignoring the child's need for necessary services and interventions

The definition of psychological abuse used in this guide combines the Hart, Brassard, and Karlson (1996), Hart, Brassard, Binggeli et al. (2002), and the NIS-3 (Sedlack and Broadhurst, 1996) definitions, but omits items such as mental heath, medical, and educational neglect and other behaviors subsumed under the neglect definitions to follow. Thus, *psychological abuse* is defined here as including the following:

1. Verbal or emotional assault, exemplified by persistent patterns of belittling, denigrating, scapegoating, or other nonphysical but rejecting, hostile, and degrading behaviors
2. Terrorizing the child, exemplified by threatening to physically hurt, kill, or abandon the child, or by exposing the child to chronic or extreme partner abuse or other forms of violent behaviors
3. Exploiting or corrupting the child, exemplified by modeling criminal or antisocial behavior; encouraging and condoning delinquent behavior, substance abuse, or other maladaptive acts; or by promoting developmentally inappropriate behaviors
4. Isolating the child, exemplified by placing unreasonable limits or restrictions on the child's social interactions and interfering with the child's developmental needs for peer and adult social interaction
5. Punishments that involve extreme confinement such as tying or binding a child, confining a child to a restrictive area such as a closet or a basement, or excessive, prolonged confinement
6. Other psychological abuses include withholding shelter, sleep, or other necessities as punishment; economic exploitation; at-

tempted sexual or physical assaults; and intentionally disregarding the child's needs for love and affection and denying emotional responsiveness

Neglect

In addition to abuse, child maltreatment evaluations also involve the assessment of neglect. The NIS-3 (Sedlack and Broadhurst, 1996) defined neglect as failing to care for the child's physical, emotional, and educational needs. Barnett and colleagues (1994) include failing to provide not only for the child's academic education but also for the child's social and moral education. This latter category included behaviors such as exposing a child to or involving a child in illegal activities and behaviors that were included in the psychological abuse category previously described.

The majority of behaviors described in the NIS-3 and by Barnett and colleagues' neglect categories include failures to recognize or respond to a child's developmental needs. As such, neglect typically involves acts of omission rather than commission. Thus, the assessment of neglect often requires determining what is missing rather than what is occurring. *Neglect* is defined in this guide as involving two categories: physical neglect and psychological neglect, both of which are detailed as follows.

Physical Neglect

Barnett and colleagues (1994) defined neglect as failing to provide for a child's physical requirements, including nutrition, health, medical, or cleanliness needs. They also defined neglect as failing to provide adequate precautions to assure a child's safety within or outside the home and failing to provide adequate supervision that is commensurate with the child's developmental needs.

In accordance with the NIS-3 (Sedlack and Broadhurst, 1996) definition and consistent with the definition offered by Barnett and colleagues, *physical neglect* will be defined in this guide as including the following actions or inactions:

1. The failure to provide reasonable medical care that is recommended by health care professionals

2. Failing to seek timely and appropriate medical services for serious health problems that would be recognizable as requiring medical attention by most laypersons
3. Not attending to a child's need for food, adequate clothing, hygiene, and immunizations
4. Disregarding safety hazards
5. Not adequately supervising the child as a result of drunkenness, drug abuse, or psychiatric disorders
6. Leaving a child in the care of an inadequate "caregiver," such as someone with a history of child abuse, and failing to protect a child by permitting abusive people to have access to the child
7. Abandoning a child or expelling a child from the home without arranging for reasonable care and supervision
8. Repeatedly leaving a child with others for extended periods in a manner suggesting a dereliction of parental custodial responsibilities
9. Leaving a child unsupervised or inadequately supervised

Psychological Neglect

The definition of *psychological neglect* used in the guide incorporates the NIS-3 (Sedlack and Broadhurst, 1996) emotional and educational neglect categories. As such, psychological neglect by a parent or caregiver may be evidenced by the following:

1. Inadequate nurturing and affection
2. Not opposing a child's substance abuse
3. Not opposing or permitting other problem behaviors such as assaultive behavior or chronic delinquency and, when aware of the problem, not attempting to intervene
4. Failing to seek or provide needed treatment for a child's emotional or behavioral problems that would be recognizable as requiring professional attention by most laypersons (such as severe depression or a suicide attempt)
5. Failure to facilitate needed psychological treatment for a child's emotional or behavioral difficulties as reasonably recommended by a qualified professional
6. Not attending to additional developmental and emotional needs not previously described such as by engaging in behaviors that foster immaturity or emotional overdependence, or by continu-

ous, inappropriate expectations for the child's age or developmental level

7. Failing to oppose or permitting chronic truancy
8. Failing to enroll a child in school, causing a child to miss school excessively (at least one month), or causing or permitting a child to stay home for nonlegitimate reasons for an average of at least three days a month (numerical parameters as set forth by the NIS-3, Sedlack and Broadhurst, 1996)
9. Failure to obtain recommended special education services or treatment for a child's diagnosed learning disorder or special education needs without reasonable cause

The definition of psychological neglect used in this guide differs from the NIS-3 in one important area. NIS-3 defines exposing a child to intrafamilial violence as psychological neglect. The present authors have classified exposure to intrafamilial violence as psychological abuse rather than psychological neglect. Although we agree that when children are exposed to such acts their needs are being neglected, it is our hypothesis that the psychological trauma inflicted as a result of witnessing intrafamilial violence is closer to the negative effects that children suffer from other forms of abuse. This position is consistent with Jaffe and colleagues (1990), who found that, for some children, witnessing partner abuse might be just as harmful to the child's healthy development as being a victim of violence. Consequently, exposure to intrafamilial violence is included as a form of psychological abuse.

When assessing physical and psychological neglect, a parent's refusal of specific medical, psychological, or educational services may require careful evaluation. When such refusal occurs as the result of cultural or religious beliefs and in the context of an otherwise nonabusive and nonneglecting relationship, the act of refusal by itself may not constitute child neglect.

In conclusion, as previously noted, the definitions of child maltreatment provided in this guide, and the examples of physical abuse, sexual abuse, psychological abuse, physical neglect, and psychological neglect given herein, are provided to facilitate clinical assessments involving child maltreatment. They are not intended to be a list of behaviors that determine whether or not a particular act is evidence of child maltreatment. They are provided to assist clinicians in becoming better at identifying and articulating behaviors that can and do cause harm to children, and to facilitate the clinician's abilities to identify causative factors and develop appropriate clinical interventions. The ultimate utility of these definitions as a classification scheme requires further investigation.

Chapter 2

The Impact of Child Maltreatment

In his 1996 commentary on the definition of family violence and family maltreatment, Geffner wrote that the effect of maltreatment on victims, in general, would be to produce "trauma." This theoretical observation is consistent with the increasingly large body of controlled, scientific research supporting the general conclusion that child maltreatment is, in fact, associated with the development of both short-term and long-term negative psychosocial outcomes in child victims. Although these studies vary in scientific rigor, and some topics, such as child neglect, are infrequently studied, the available literature does indicate that child maltreatment is associated with trauma and that children who suffer various forms of child maltreatment often experience negative effects on their behavioral, emotional, and cognitive adjustment.

However, before discussing the possible symptoms associated with child maltreatment, a cautionary remark is in order. It must be emphasized that no specific behavioral symptom exhibited by a child can be assumed to indicate that the child was abused or neglected in a particular manner or, for that matter, that the child was abused or neglected at all. For example, it is widely believed that sexual behavior problems in children indicate that they were sexually abused. However, a recent study of children referred for sexual abuse evaluations found that the presence versus absence of sexual behavior problems did not predict whether the child has been abused (Drach et al., 2001). Rather, alternative hypotheses are often necessary to account for the presence of such behavior problems. Furthermore, studies of children who have not been sexually abused have identified multiple variables associated with sexual behavioral problems, such as family nudity, life stress, and exposure to domestic violence (Friedrich et al., 1991, 1998). In addition, one study of children with sexual behavior problems (Gray et al., 1997) found a relationship between domestic violence and sexual behavior. Thus, in child maltreatment evaluations, as is the case in other types of child mental health evaluations, a particular type of behavior problem may have multiple alternative etiologies.

With this caution in mind, and as previously noted, child maltreatment has been shown to be generally associated with a range of negative outcomes. Some of these outcomes may be acute, others may be lasting. Lasting effects may significantly affect the child's development in a number of ways. As Berliner (1997) observed,

> children's biochemistry, information processing, and memory may be altered in significant ways; children who cannot concentrate or dissociate may fall behind at school; children who constrict emotional responses or who do not learn to regulate negative abuse-related affects may not develop the capacity to experience the full range of emotions or engage in satisfying interpersonal relationships; and children who feel stigmatized or cannot cope with the reactions of others may avoid peers or interact in inappropriate ways. (p. 161)

The existing research also shows that the negative effects of child maltreatment may continue into adulthood and become associated with various forms of adult social, psychological, and psychiatric maladjustment (Banyard, 1999; Berenbaum, 1999; Johnson et al., 1999; Neumann et al., 1996; Miller and Lisak, 1999; Mullen et al., 1996; Weeks and Widom, 1998; Widom, 1999). This chapter summarizes the research relating to the negative and traumatic impact of child maltreatment.

THE IMPACT OF CHILD MALTREATMENT ON ATTACHMENT SECURITY

Attachment theory maintains that infants are born with a survival-based drive to seek proximity to and safety from primary caregivers during times of emotional distress. The repeated experience of successfully regaining a sense of security from attachment figures is a prerequisite to the development of secure attachments.

Research studies have increasingly found that attachment difficulties are associated with problems in affect regulation, behavioral controls, and interpersonal difficulties beginning in early childhood, and that these difficulties may extend through adolescence and adulthood (Bates and Bayles, 1988; Carlson, 1998; Dutton, 1995; Fonagy et al., 1996; Greenberg and Speltz, 1988; Jacobvitz and Hazen, 1999; Lyons-Ruth, 1996; Moss et al., 1999; Rosenstein and Horowitz, 1996; Rubin and Lollis, 1988; van IJzendoorn and Bakermans-Kranenburg, 1996). For example, Cicchetti and Toth (1995) noted that difficulties in the development of attachment security might negatively affect self/other differentiation, peer relationships, and the development of intimate relationships. Secure attachments are considered fundamental for children to develop the ability to regulate disorganizing emotions such as anxiety and fear. When the infant's ability to establish attachment security is compromised, the child's ability to learn to trust or develop relationships based on reciprocity and empathy is jeopardized. Research has demonstrated that child maltreatment is a significant risk factor for attachment insecurity and associated relationship disturbances (Carlson, 1998; Carlson et al., 1989; Cicchetti et al., 1995; Crittenden, 1988; Lynch and Cicchetti, 1991; Main and Solomon, 1990; Schuengel et al., 1999). In the absence of secure attachments, maltreated children become increasingly more at risk than nonmaltreated children for failing to learn how to effectively manage their feelings and behaviors. As such, child maltreatment is an important risk factor for significant attachment-related emotional and behavioral problems across the life span.

THE IMPACT OF PHYSICAL ABUSE

Controlled research studies have repeatedly demonstrated that physical abuse is a powerful psychosocial risk factor for children in a variety of areas of functioning. As a result of physical abuse, children may experience medical injuries that are acute or lasting (Kolko, 2002). In addition, studies have shown that, compared with non-abused children, physically abused children evidence more signs of emotional disturbance, especially internalizing emotional problems such as anxiety and depression (de Paúl and Arruabarrena, 1995; Jaffe et al., 1986; Kaufman, 1991; Kolko, 1992; Lizardi et al., 1995;

Toth et al., 1992). Physically abused children also demonstrate more externalizing behavioral problems than nonabused children do. These behaviors include increased aggressive behavior, conduct problems, and peer relationship difficulties (Jaffe et al., 1986; Kolko, 1992; Knutson, 1995). In addition, physically abused children have been found to exhibit more developmental deficits than their nonabused peers, including decreased intelligence and more academic performance difficulties (Kolko, 1992; de Paúl and Arruabarrena, 1995). Finally, physically abused children are more likely than nonabused children to experience attachment difficulties (Kolko, 1992).

A variety of studies also have found that the long-term effects of child physical abuse may include depression, suicidal and self-injurious behaviors, and other emotional disorders in adolescence and adulthood (Lizardi et al., 1995). Long-term effects of child physical abuse may also include decreased intelligence (Perez and Widom, 1994), psychological and psychiatric difficulties (Malinosky-Rummell and Hansen, 1993), intimacy problems (Ducharme et al., 1997), and attitudes and behaviors supporting the use of physical discipline, criminality, and familial and nonfamilial forms of violence (Bowker et al., 1988; Malinosky-Rummell and Hansen, 1993; Widom, 1989).

THE IMPACT OF SEXUAL ABUSE

Literature reviews of research studies on the effects of sexual abuse (Briere and Elliott, 1994; Browne and Finkelhor, 1986; Kendall-Tackett et al., 1993) have indicated that sexually abused children are more likely than nonabused children to exhibit emotional distress such as anxiety, phobias, depression, embarrassment, anger, and posttraumatic stress disorders. Feelings of powerlessness, helplessness, shame, and guilt may contribute to a distorted sense of self and a diinished sense of self-esteem and self-worth. In addition, in comparison to nonabused children, sexually abused children more frequently experience an inadequate sense of self, feelings of betrayal, and difficulties in the area of interpersonal trust that contribute to increased attachment difficulties, social isolation, and interpersonal problems. Sexually abused children experience increased rates of psychosomatic and physiological symptoms, including bed-wetting, sleep disturbances, and somatic complaints. Higher rates of tension-reducing behaviors have been observed and may include dissociation, substance abuse, eating disorders, sexual behavior problems, and antisocial behaviors (Browne and Finkelhor, 1986; Briere and Elliott, 1994; Friedrich et al., 1992; Friedrich, 1993; Kendall-Tackett et al., 1993).

Research on the long-term effects of childhood sexual abuse has also documented a variety of serious psychological and social problems. These problems include substance abuse, depression, suicidal thoughts and actions, self-mutilating behaviors, eating disorders, alcohol and drug addiction, adult attachment difficulties and chronic relationship problems, and experiencing various forms of revictimization in adulthood (Becker et al., 1995; Briere and Elliott, 1994; DiLillo and Long, 1999; Messman-Moore and Long, 2000; Neumann et al., 1996; Perez and Widom, 1994; Roche et al., 1999). In addition, sexual abuse has been associated with increased sexual difficulties, such as aversions to intimate relationships, sexual dysfunction, sexual identity confusion, sexualized behavior, and sexual revictimization (Becker and Hunter, 1997; Browne and Finkelhor, 1986; Briere and Elliott, 1994; Friedrich, 1993; Messman-Moore and Long, 2000; Neumann et al., 1996; Tyler et al., 2000).

THE IMPACT OF PSYCHOLOGICAL MALTREATMENT

Becker and her colleagues (1995) have noted that psychological maltreatment is a difficult area to study empirically because of significant problems in defining what it is and because psychological maltreatment typically co-occurs with other forms of child maltreatment. These authors concluded, however, that available research indicates that psychological maltreatment, in isolation or in combination with other forms of abuse, is associated with a range of psychosocial problems beyond those generally found among children from disadvantaged environments.

Verbal abuse involving parents swearing at, insulting, and being verbally aggressive toward their children has been found to have severe negative psychosocial consequences for children. For example, parental verbal aggression toward children has been associated with increased physically aggressive behaviors, delinquency, and social problems, as well as negative effects on academic achievement and self-esteem (Solomon and Serres, 1999; Vissing et al., 1991). Also, Dutton and colleagues (1995) found that childhood shaming experiences such as public scolding, random punishment, and criticism affecting the child's sense of self were associated with increased rates of partner violence in adulthood. This finding remained strong even when the data analysis controlled for the experience of physically abusive experiences during childhood.

Psychological maltreatment can occur in the absence of other forms of child maltreatment but more commonly happens in conjunction with other forms of abuse or neglect (Claussen and Crittenden, 1991). The negative effects of psychological maltreatment on children's adjustment appear, however, to be substantial, independent from the effects of the co-occurring forms of maltreatment (McGee et al., 1997), and psychological maltreatment potentially is responsible for more negative effects on children than physical abuse alone (Crittenden, 1996). Perhaps, as Crittenden reported, psychological abuse or maltreatment is "an insidious component" inherent to all types of child abuse.

THE IMPACT OF EXPOSURE TO FAMILY VIOLENCE

Research studies demonstrate that exposing children to family violence may have serious consequences for the psychosocial development of children, even when children are not directly abused (Edleson, 1999a; Jaffe et al., 1992; Kolbo et al., 1996; O'Keefe, 1994; Miller-Perrin and Perrin, 1999). Exposure as defined here follows Edleson's definition and includes the child's seeing the abuse, hearing it, and being used symbolically as a weapon by the perpetrator.

The studies (Fantuzzo et al., 1991; Jaffe et al., 1986; Jouriles and Norwood, 1995; Shipman et al., 1999; Sternberg et al., 1993) indicate that children who are exposed to family maltreatment manifest more depression and anxiety than do their nonexposed peers. They also demonstrate increased behavioral problems such as disobedience, lying and cheating, fighting, destruction of property, and peer relationship difficulties. In addition, boys who are exposed to partner violence, in particular, have been found to engage in higher rates of dating violence (O'Keefe, 1997).

Children who are exposed to partner abuse frequently have been found to lack adequate safety skills to cope with violent incidents and be more likely to condone violence as a means of resolving conflict (Jaffe et al., 1988). For some children, witnessing partner abuse may be just as harmful to the child's healthy development as being the one abused (Jaffe et al., 1990) and the effects may last into adulthood (Henning et al., 1996; Silvern et al., 1995).

As noted in the Preface, although child maltreatment research provides increased understanding of factors associated with child abuse and neglect, because of methodological difficulties, findings must be evaluated cautiously. Caution is especially warranted in the area of children's exposure to partner violence (Edleson, 1999a; Miller-Perrin and Perrin, 1999). Special problems in this area of research include assumed exposure to partner violence without actual documentation when children live with adults who have engaged in partner violence. In addition, studies frequently use samples of mothers and children at battered women's shelters. These subjects may not be representative of a more inclusive population of children exposed to partner violence and their responses may be inaccurate or skewed, for example, by high levels of situational stress.

THE IMPACT OF NEGLECT

There are a limited number of studies focusing specifically on the impact of physical and psychological neglect on child development. Poverty and child neglect are highly correlated, however research findings have documented that the potential negative effects of child neglect on children extend beyond those problems and difficulties that can be attributed to poverty (Gaudin, 1999; Crittenden, 1999).

Available studies suggest that neglected children are more likely than other children to exhibit delays in language, intellectual development, and academic achievement (Crouch and Milner, 1993; Gaudin, 1999). Neglected children also may experience more attachment and peer relationship difficulties, emotional and behavioral problems, coping difficulties, and may have higher levels of psychopathology than children who are not maltreated (Crouch and Milner, 1993). As this review indicates, however, children who experience other forms of maltreatment may experience these difficulties as well.

Crittenden (1996) noted that neglected children often become increasingly listless and apathetic. As the children become more passive, they may provide fewer cues to their parents for engagement, which in turn may contribute to an interactive cycle of less stimulation and further neglect. Yet, while many neglected children show a pattern of passivity and depression, some react by becoming extremely active, seeming to be "frantic in their seeking of stimulation" (Crittenden, 1996, p. 163). Ongoing problems can include attachment difficulties, peer relationship difficulties, and decreased prosocial behavior when compared with other children (Becker et al., 1995; Crouch and Milner, 1993; Knutson, 1995).

Egeland (1997) described a group of emotionally neglected children whose parents were psychologically unavailable. These parents were characterized as emotionally detached and uninvolved with their children. They typically interacted with their children only when it appeared essential and they did not seem to engage with their children emotionally or enjoy caring for them. Egeland (1993) reported that he and his colleagues have found that this kind of maltreatment has pernicious effects on young children's development. Children of psychologically unavailable parents were observed to be insecurely attached at eighteen months, displaying more negative affect than nonmaltreated controls at twenty-four months, and showing more negative, oppositional, and avoidant behaviors at forty-two months (Egeland, 1997). Multiple regression analyses conducted as part of this longitudinal, prospective study indicated that psychological unavailability in early childhood was a strong predictor of adolescent onset aggression in children. When combined with sexual abuse victimization and other forms of neglect, psychological unavailability also predicted delinquency in adolescence.

THE IMPACT OF MULTIPLE FORMS OF CHILD MALTREATMENT

One factor complicating research into the sequelae of specific types of child abuse and neglect is the fact that different forms of maltreatment frequently co-occur (Barnett et al., 1994; McGee et al., 1997; Ney et al., 1994). Individual children often are victims of multiple forms of abuse, either directly or as a witness to the abuse of siblings or a parent. McGee and colleagues (1995) found that 36 percent of the adolescents in their study had experienced four of five types of maltreatment. Twenty percent had experienced them all. Only 6.3 percent of the youths had experienced just one form of maltreatment.

Existing studies of the impact of combinations of child abuse and neglect (Mullen et al., 1996; Ney et al., 1994) indicate that some combinations of maltreatment, such as the combination of physical neglect, physical abuse, and verbal abuse, are associated with more malignant outcomes than are others. Further research is needed, however, to more fully delineate this important issue.

COMPARATIVE STUDIES OF THE IMPACT OF ABUSE AND NEGLECT

Most research studies of the impact of child maltreatment do not distinguish between or compare types of abuse and neglect. When comparative analyses have been conducted, many similarities between groups have been found (Jaffe et al., 1986; Mullen et al., 1996). Some differences in the negative effects of different forms of maltreatment also have been observed. For example, Toth et al. (1992) found that children who had been physically abused exhibited significantly higher levels of depressive symptoms than either physically neglected or nonmaltreated children. Other findings (Mullen et al., 1996) suggest that children who have been sexually abused may develop increased levels of sexual problems than those who have been physically abused, but that emotionally abused children also may experience sexual difficulties. In spite of such group differences, research clearly demonstrates that children who have been maltreated, either singly or in combination, are at risk for experiencing negative effects throughout their lives as a result of the maltreatment. Table 2.1 provides a summary of research findings reflecting the negative impact of child maltreatment.

THE IMPACT OF MARGINAL MALTREATMENT

According to NIS findings, child protective service agencies investigate less than half of received reports of child abuse (Sedlack and Broadhurst, 1996). Of the cases investigated, half may be closed following initial investigation. Many of the families in these cases have been described as exhibiting marginal forms of maltreatment (Crittenden, 1996). In such cases child-rearing problems exist and may be

TABLE 2.1. Impact of Child Abuse and Neglect

Area of Functioning	Clinical Examples
Cognitive	Problems in academic learning, such as may be reflected in school failure and lower cognitive skills; for example, difficulties in problem solving or using cognitive skills to delay or modulate emotion. Failure to internalize the cognitive components of conscience (knowing what is right and wrong). Lower IQ.
Emotional	Problems in emotional regulation; for example, impulsivity, excessive fears and anxiety, and other emotional difficulties. Post-traumatic stress disorder and mood disorders. Defects in empathy.
Self-Image and Self-Concept	Distorted self-image, such as views self as worthless and inadequate, low self-esteem, distorted body image.
Behavioral	Problems in behavioral functioning, such as conduct problems (e.g., impulsive, sensation-seeking, and antisocial behaviors), substance abuse, and so on.
Interpersonal	Disordered attachment behaviors, such as avoidant or conflicted patterns of attachment insecurity when distressed, an inability to secure comforting from caretakers, responding to a crying peer with aggression, and so on. Aggressive behaviors (verbal, passive-aggressive, physical). Failure to develop effective social skills. Association with asocial, deviant, or antisocial peers.
Psychophysiological	Failure to thrive, poor appetite, encopresis or enuresis, other somatic manifestations, such as headaches, stomachaches, and so on.

Problems in Socialization and the Acquisition of Prosocial Attitudes	Defects in socialization and moral reasoning. Problems in social learning, such as distorted perceptual accuracy in social situations (i.e., distortion of incoming data by one's own expectations, attitudes, and beliefs), negative attributions, not learning the rules of appropriate social behavior (such as through defective modeling and exposure to inaccurate information). Asocial, deviant, or antisocial cognitive distortions, such as sentiments, attitudes, beliefs, and values that justify maltreatment or antisocial behavior.

accompanied by low levels of abuse and neglect, but they are not considered severe enough to warrant state intervention.

In spite of such determinations, the psychosocial impact of marginal maltreatment may be significant. For example, Herman (1981) found that daughters of sexually seductive fathers experienced significant psychological difficulties that were similar in type, although not in severity, to girls who were described as having been sexually abused.

THE IMPACT OF MEDIATING FACTORS

The effects of child maltreatment vary over time and among children. Although negative effects often are associated with child maltreatment, some children appear to be less affected than others and, in some cases, child victims may not manifest any symptoms associated with their experiences of child maltreatment. For example, in Kendall-Tackett and colleagues' (1993) review of forty-five studies of children who had been sexually abused, between 21 percent and 49 percent had no symptoms suggesting they had been maltreated.

The impact of child abuse and neglect in any given case may depend, in part, upon factors specific to the maltreatment. These factors include the type of maltreatment, its frequency, duration, and the presence of combined types of maltreatment in a given case (Alksnis and Taylor, 1994; Bennett et al., 2000; Edleson, 1999a; Manly et al., 1994; Ney et al., 1994; Perez and Widom, 1994; Wind and Silvern, 1992). For example, force or violence and victim injury have been associated with increased negative effects in victims of child sexual abuse (Browne and Finkelhor, 1986; Gomes-Schwartz et al., 1990). Similarly, more invasive forms of sexual abuse have been associated with more severe outcomes (Bennett et al., 2000; Mennen and Meadow, 1995).

The child's relationship with the perpetrator also may increase the trauma, for example, when the perpetrator is a trusted family member or biological parent (Berliner and Elliott, 2002; Briere and Elliott, 1994; Sullivan et al., 2000; Wind and Silvern, 1992). In addition, high levels of stress and parental psychopathology have been associated with negative outcomes for children who have been abused (Deblinger et al., 1999; Wind and Silvern, 1994).

Wind and Silvern (1994), however, found that although high family stress was associated with childhood histories of abuse and psychological problems in adulthood, parental support mediated the relationship between childhood abuse and subsequent negative effects. High family stress was not a risk factor for negative outcomes in adulthood when parental warmth and support was experienced. In addition, factors such as family cohesiveness and stability (Mullen et al., 1996; Ray and Jackson, 1997; Wolfe, 1994); positive parenting and parental modeling of resilience (Herrenkohl et al., 1991); and positive intrafamilial and extrafamilial social supports (Banyard, 1999; Deblinger et al., 1999; Everson et al., 1989; Feiring et al., 1998; Mannarino and Cohen, 1996; McMillen and Zuravin, 1997), such as a good relationship with a grandparent (Grizenko and Pawliuk, 1994), may help buffer the negative effects of maltreatment.

Other factors that may mediate the effects of child maltreatment include the developmental stage of the child at the time of the maltreatment. Finkelhor (1997) observed:

> For example, young children victimized at an early age by their primary caretakers seem to suffer a big developmental impact in the form of insecure attachments to caregivers . . . Children victimized during preschool years, when children experiment with normal dissociative skills, may be those who become most likely to use dissociation as a defense mechanism and to develop a pattern of dissociation that becomes chronic . . . And sexual abuse and other trauma can hasten the onset of puberty. . . . (p. 103)

Increasingly, neurodevelopmental research (Glaser, 2000; Schwarz and Perry, 1994) suggests that child abuse and neglect can affect brain development at critical and sensitive periods; consequently, child maltreatment may have lasting effects on a child's cognitive, emotional, behavioral, and interpersonal functioning (Glaser, 2000).

Personal factors that may influence the effects of child maltreatment include the individual's personal adjustment (O'Keefe, 1994), the child's level of intellectual functioning (Herrenkohl et al., 1991; Herrenkohl et al., 1994), the ability to express feelings (Grizenko and Pawliuk, 1994), whether the child has a more internalized or externalized locus of control (Banyard, 1999; Herrenkohl et al., 1994; Mannarino and Cohen, 1996), and whether the child has special interests, such as multiple hobbies (Grizenko and Pawliuk, 1994). Additional factors involve the child's cognitive appraisals and attributions pertaining to the maltreatment, such as feelings of self-blame and stigmatization (Coffey et al., 1996; Finkelhor, 1997; Kuehnle, 1996; Mannarino and Cohen, 1996; McMillen and Zuravin, 1997).

Such findings are consistent with research investigating children considered to be at high risk for negative outcomes due to biological and psychosocial risk factors, such as perinatal stress and adverse rearing conditions (Werner, 1989). Werner followed children born in Hawaii in 1955 for a thirty-year period and found that subjects who were classified as resilient were seen from childhood as good-natured and tended to have more interests and hobbies, a positive self-concept, and internal locus of control.

Mullen and colleagues (1996) pointed out that it is possible that other risk factors associated with child maltreatment and its effects, such as parental discord, family instability, and not having a confiding mother-child relationship, may account for many of the reported mental health and interpersonal difficulties, independent of child maltreatment. They investigated this possibility and found that such difficulties in adulthood are related to varied risk factors and that the effects of child maltreatment were modest. Such findings highlight the importance of assessing a range of risk factors that may be associated with the negative effects of child maltreatment on individuals and the perpetuation of intergenerational cycles of maltreatment, as well as other forms of social disadvantage and developmental influences, and then intervening accordingly.

Egeland and his colleagues (1988) conducted a study designed to distinguish characteristics of mothers who had been abused as children but who did not abuse their own children as contrasted with those who did abuse their children. They found:

> Abused mothers who were able to break the abusive cycle were significantly more likely to have received emotional support from a nonabusive adult during childhood, participated in therapy during any period of their lives, and to have had a nonabusive and more stable, emotionally supportive, and satisfying relationship with a mate. Abused mothers who reenacted their maltreatment with their own children experienced significantly more life stress and were more anxious, dependent, immature, and depressed. (p. 1080)

These findings are consistent with Egeland's subsequent review of research findings from the child maltreatment and child development literature (1993, 1997). He found a number of variables that may serve to protect against or mitigate the impact of child maltreatment. These factors include the following:

1. Past developmental history of competence
2. Secure attachment in infancy
3. The availability of a supportive caregiver or other emotionally supportive individuals during childhood or adolescence
4. A stable, predictable, and organized home environment
5. A stable family situation
6. A high quality preschool or school setting that is well organized and supportive
7. Having integrated the abusive experience into their experience of themselves, in contrast with idealizing or dissociating the past

The variability and diversity in outcomes for maltreated children may also be related, in part, to a number of other factors such as poverty, family stress, chaotic and disorganized home environments, and the interaction of maltreatment and other related risk factors (Egeland, 1997; Widom, 1999). However, the negative effects of child maltreatment also are independent of such varied difficulties and cannot, therefore, be simply discounted. As Egeland (1997) stressed based on follow-ups of the children who were studied, "Some maltreated children were doing better than others, but none were invulnerable to the negative consequences of early maltreatment" (p. 14).

Chapter 3

Risk Assessment

PROBLEMS AND STRATEGIES FOR ASSESSING VIOLENCE

A review of the literature on family maltreatment and sexual violence (Righthand et al., 1998) revealed that most factors associated with serious forms of child maltreatment also are associated with interpersonal violence in general. The professional literature discussed in Chapter 2 illustrated that, as with other forms of violence, child maltreatment can harm, injure, and traumatize victims and the negative sequelae of maltreatment can have lifelong effects (Cicchetti and Toth, 1995). Considering the actual or potential consequences of child maltreatment, it appears fair to say that, as Emery and Laumann-Billings (1998) have noted, "What we have called maltreatment may be on a continuum of what we have termed violence, [and] . . . acts of abuse may differ from normal family aggression only by a matter of degree" (p. 131). The linking of child maltreatment to the larger issue of violence enables those working in the "family maltreatment" (p. 3) field to make use of the substantial body of theory and research regarding human aggression and interpersonal violence to better understand issues related to child maltreatment and further inform assessments and interventions (Geffner, 1996).

One of the key findings in the literature pertaining to human aggression and interpersonal violence is that violence is very difficult to predict. Research critiquing the accuracy of clinical assessments and predictions of violence span more than two decades (Monahan, 1981). Early studies revealed those empirical attempts at prediction failed significantly (Monahan and Steadman, 1994).

Subsequent work in this area has demonstrated that attempts at prediction have failed because violence is a rare event, and rare events are inherently difficult to predict because of what is known as the base rate problem. Put simply, if an event occurs one time in one hundred thousand, it is very easy to predict that this event will not occur, but it is exceptionally difficult to predict the one time in one hundred thousand that it will occur. Consequently, prediction is the wrong strategy.

More recently, researchers have addressed this question by adopting a new strategy, referred to as risk assessment (Monahan and Steadman, 1994). In contrast to prediction models that attempt to specify whether or not an event will occur, a risk assessment model seeks to identify specific factors that either increase or mitigate risk. Thus, the risk assessment model does not result in a dichotomous prediction of occurrence or nonoccurrence.

Even with the transition from predictive models to risk assessment models, the most recent research still suggests the validity of unassisted clinical judgments of violence "are modest at best. Computer software that may enable improved, statistically complex, risk assessment approaches appear on the horizon for individuals with mental disorders" (The MacArthur Violence Risk Assessment Study, 2001, p. 1). These sophisticated approaches may lead to improvements in risk assessment with other populations as well. In the meantime, despite current risk assessment limitations, the social, legal, and political demands for accurate predictions persist (Limandri and Seridan, 1995), largely because violence, as well as the erroneous prediction of violence, has severe consequences for victims, family members, and the community. Thus, ethical and scientific discussions about how best to approach this difficult task are relevant (Borum, 1996; Grisso and Appelbaum, 1992; Webster et al., 1994).

It is beyond the scope of this guide to discuss in detail the wealth of data encompassing the clinical, legal, and ethical issues concerning violence prediction and risk assessment. Clinicians who conduct risk assessments should be well acquainted with this literature base and the difficulties inherent in this work (see Limandri and Seridan, 1995; Melton et al., 1997; Monahan, 1981; Quinsey et al., 1998; Webster et al., 1997b).

The application of risk assessment strategies to the field of child maltreatment is a relatively new area of study. Because the course of human development is complex and interactive with situational and environmental influences, risk assessment in cases of child abuse and neglect must consider multiple factors. Assessment strategies that focus on too few variables or single points in time will tend to decrease the reliability and validity of the risk assessment (Daro, 1996; Milner, 1995).

Further complicating this issue is the multidimensional nature of child maltreatment. Although some researchers (e.g., Barbaree and Marshall, 1988; Milner, 1995) have focused exclusively on specific types of child maltreatment, most research has failed to distinguish between the various categories of child abuse and neglect. This chapter will look at the risk factors for distinct types whenever possible. The research to date, however, suggests that risk and protective factors are frequently consistent across multiple types of maltreatment.

The most sophisticated risk assessment research effort to date is the MacArthur Violence Risk Assessment Study (2001). Noting the methodological shortcomings of existing studies, this project sought to improve upon previous research in a variety of ways. For example, researchers emphasized the importance of defining a "large and diverse array of risk factors" (p. 2). They began by reviewing existing studies of violence and mental disorders and found potentially robust variables that could prove useful for assessing violence among people with mental disorders. They classified the selected variables into four areas: (1) dispositional factors; (2) historical or developmental factors; (3) contextual or situational variables; and (4) clinical or specific symptom factors, and used sophisticated statistical procedures to investigate the utility of these variables in a multisite study of persons with mental disorders.

The advantages and limitations of various risk assessment approaches are discussed in Chapter 5. This chapter will utilize the format employed in the MacArthur Violence Risk Assessment Study (2001) to identify the static (unchanging) and dynamic (changing) variables that have been empirically related to the risk of child maltreatment and are relevant for child maltreatment risk assessments. The assessment areas are presented here in a different sequence than described in the MacArthur study in order to facilitate clinical assessments.

1. Historical or developmental factors
2. Dispositional or personal factors
3. Clinical or symptom factors
4. Contextual or situation variables

Risk assessment is best conducted by examining verbal and behavioral evidence across time and situations. Likely sources of information include records, observations, interviews, and psychological testing, along with collateral contacts and corroborating data. Although an increased number of risk factors may be associated with a greater risk of maltreatment (Brown et al., 1998; Marshall and English, 1999), in some cases even one or two may be critical (Webster et al., 1997b).

As will be discussed in Chapter 5, when conducting risk assessments, base rate information detailing the prevalence of characteristics or behaviors in a population is a very important starting point for enhancing accuracy and reducing biases. Unfortunately, base rate information may not always be available. For example, DePanfilis and Zuravin (1998) reviewed available studies pertaining to child maltreatment reoccurrences. They reported that existing studies pertaining to child maltreatment recidivism are limited in number and by methodological difficulties. They cautioned that specific conclusions pertaining to the base rate of child maltreatment recidivism are premature and recommended that, at a minimum, trends within communities or states be identified and methodologically sound prospective research with adequate sample sizes be conducted. DePanfilis and Zuravin did note that the available research findings suggested that the risk of reoccurrence was higher among families who experienced multiple types of maltreatment and that

> . . . with the exception of recurrence rates for groups of CPS [Child Protective Services] families deemed to be at low risk of future maltreatment, CPS agencies nationally may be serving a significant percentage of their population over and over again. (p. 36)

In contrast to the field of child abuse and neglect, research focusing on sex offense recidivism appears somewhat more advanced. For example, Hanson and Bussière's (1998) metaanalytic results indicate that the known recidivism rate for sexual offending averaged 13.4 percent based upon studies that on average had four- to five-year follow-up periods. Some subgroups of sex offenders reoffended at higher rates, however, such as extrafamilial offenders and those who sexually assaulted adult victims. Hanson and Bussière cautioned that the findings of their studies should be interpreted cautiously because of the divergent methodology between studies included in the analysis and because many sexual offenses are undetected (Bonta and Hanson as cited in Hanson and Bussière). They noted that higher rates of recidivism have been found in studies with especially thorough record searches and long follow-up periods, yet they observed that, even with these procedures, reoffense rates rarely exceeded 40 percent.

Professionals frequently are required to identify short-term predictors of maltreatment. Unfortunately, limited research is available on this topic. Fluke and colleagues (2001) investigated the effectiveness of a child protective safety protocol for reducing short-term recurrence of maltreatment. The protocol included items that were "readily observable, immediate, and harmful" (p. 208), such as current violent or out of control behavior, the presence of extremely negative attitudes or unrealistic expectations involving the child, and persistent inability to provide supervision necessary to prevent the possibility of serious harm. Fluke found that in spite of the very low base rate of short-term recurrences of maltreatment (defined as recurrences within sixty days), the short-term recurrence of maltreatment was significantly reduced after the implementation of the safety protocol. Alternative explanations for the reduction in short-term recurrences did not appear responsible for the reduced incidence of maltreatment.

Noting the dearth of research addressing when sex offenders are most likely to reoffend, Hanson and Harris (2000) compared recidivist and nonrecidivist sex offenders on dynamic or changeable risk factors. In spite of attempts to match the groups on relevant static or historical variables, the recidivist group had a greater history of sexual deviance and antisocial lifestyles. However, the recidivist group also demonstrated more problems while under community supervision as evidenced by poor social supports, increased attitudes tolerant of sexual assault, higher rates of antisocial behaviors, poorer self-management strategies, and greater difficulties cooperating with community supervision. Although the groups did not differ in their overall mood, those who recidivated demonstrated increased levels of anger and subjective distress just prior to re-offending. The researchers found that even after controlling for the preexisting differences, the dynamic risk factors were strongly related to recidivism. This study, as well as Fluke and colleagues' research, suggests the importance of paying attention to immediate and changeable risk factors, as well as considering more static and historical factors when considering risk.

As noted previously, many of the risk factors for child maltreatment also are risk factors for other types of violence, such as partner abuse. By and large, these risk factors reflect deficits in social competence and psychological difficulties that may be related to a cycle of intergenerational maltreatment which will continue if not identified and successfully addressed. With this point in mind, the following descriptions of relevant risk factors may serve as a useful guide for evaluating children as well as parents.

HISTORICAL OR DEVELOPMENTAL FACTORS

As used in this document, historical or developmental factors refer to events or circumstances occurring during childhood and adulthood up until the present time. Developmental and historical factors that research studies have associated with the risk of child maltreatment follow.

Family of Origin

Parental Instability During Childhood

Parental instability, as evidenced by such factors as substance abuse, mental illness, criminal behavior, frequent changes in sexual partners and household members, frequent moves or parental absences, has been associated with child maltreatment (Caplan et al., 1984; Milner and Crouch, 1993; Oates, 1997; Wolfe, 1987) and criminal behavior (Prentky and Knight, 1986). Significant parental separations or absences have been associated with general interpersonal violence (Klassen and O'Connor, 1994) and partner violence in particular (Magdol et al., 1998).

Klassen and O'Connor (1994) pointed out that parental instability and absences could disrupt adequate bonding and socialization during childhood. They noted that adequate bonding during childhood is associated with the development of empathy in adulthood, and that empathy for others is believed to be important for deterring violence against others. Perhaps consistent with this notion is Hanson and Bussière's (1998) finding that a negative relationship with the mother correlated with increased rates of sex offender sexual and general recidivism. Also supportive of this concept is the finding that reduced levels of sexual aggression in male juveniles were associated with mother-child bonding (Kobayashi et al., 1995).

Parents' Parenting Style

Another related factor associated with child maltreatment and other forms of violence is the style of parenting that the parent experienced as a child (Wolfe, 1987). Although parenting styles can vary within the course of a child's upbringing, factors such as insufficient or inadequate parental nurturing and supervision, as well as coercive or hostile parenting styles have been observed in neglectful and maltreating parents (Crittenden, 1996; Erickson and Egeland, 2002). These negative parenting styles have been associated with the development of attachment difficulties (Crittenden, 1985a; Lynch and Cicchetti, 1991) as well as delinquent and violent behavior (Klassen and O'Connor, 1994; Wolfe, 1987). Experiencing insufficient or inadequate nurturing or a coercive, hostile parenting style during childhood may, in the absence of more positive role models and supports, leave a developing child unaware of appropriate parenting behaviors and methods and may, in effect, teach maladaptive parenting behaviors.

Experience of Family Maltreatment and Family Violence During Childhood

The experience of family maltreatment and violence during childhood is a risk factor for intergenerational family maltreatment. Childhood experiences of coercive and violent family interactions are associated with the later perpetration of family violence, regardless of whether the child is directly maltreated or is only exposed to the violence (Curran, 1996; Grayson, 1995; Jones, 1987; Malinosky-Rummell and Hansen, 1993; Wolfe, 1987).

Not only have childhood experiences of child abuse and neglect been associated with maltreatment of children in adulthood but also higher rates of multiple referrals for child abuse and neglect have been found among parents who were maltreated as children (Marshall and English, 1999; English et al., 1999). It is important to note, however, that re-referrals are not the same as reoccurrences. English and colleagues (1999) reported that only about a third of referrals are substantiated at a given time. However, they also observed that the risk factors associated with multiple referrals are generally consistent with those for reoffenses.

In addition, histories of neglect as well as physical and sexual abuse have frequently been found in parents whose parental rights were terminated (Schetky et al., 1979). Childhood experiences of maltreatment also have been associated with dropping out of treatment (Jones, 1987).

Furthermore, histories of childhood maltreatment have been associated with violence and sexual violence in juveniles (Hunter and Becker, 1994; Kobayashi et al., 1995; Prentky and Knight, 1993) as well as adults (Berliner et al., 1995; Boer et al., 1997; Klassen and O'Connor, 1994; Seidman et al., 1994). Physical abuse during childhood also has been shown to be a differentiating factor between abusive husbands and controls (Rosenbaum and O'Leary, 1981). In addition, in one of the few studies that included an investigation of sibling violence, having been injured by a sibling before age fifteen predicted increased risk of violence in a sample of men admitted as inpatients at a community mental health center (Klassen and O'Connor, 1988).

As noted in Chapter 2, different forms of abuse frequently co-occur (McGee et al., 1997; Ney et al., 1994). Barnett and colleagues (1994) found that nearly 75 percent of families in their sample had experienced more than one type of maltreatment.

Widom's (1989) extensive review of the literature regarding the impact of physical abuse as a child on the later risk for physical abuse of a child estimated that 30 percent of children who were physically abused subsequently went on to abuse their own children. Due to significant methodological weaknesses in the literature, however, Widom emphasized that the differences between the abused and neglected subjects and the comparison groups were only modest and certainly could not be used as the only explanation of adult aggressive behavior. Nonetheless, from a risk assessment standpoint, a history of physical abuse during childhood has value as an indicator of increased risk (Klassen and O'Connor, 1994), as does the finding that children who are physically abused by mothers are at increased risk for persistent spousal abuse in adulthood (Aldarondo and Sugarman, 1996).

The childhood experience of sexual abuse has been associated with sexual offending in children with sexual behavior problems (e.g., Burton, 2000; Kobayashi et al., 1995; Pithers et al., 1998), as well as with adult sex offenders (e.g., Weeks and Widom, 1998). The rates vary according to sampling differences but, overall, research findings indicate that approximately 30 percent of child molesters report having been sexually abused during their childhood (Murphy and Smith, 1996). Research findings suggest that sex offenders who report sexually abusive childhood experiences tend to evidence higher levels of sexual deviancy, have increased rates of psychological disturbances, and typically come from more dysfunctional families (Murphy and Smith, 1996). Research has found that severe sexual abuse (coitus) has been associated with the intergenerational transmission of child maltreatment (Zuravin et al., 1996).

Psychological abuse also has been associated with the perpetration of child maltreatment and family violence. For example, Dutton and colleagues (1995) found that experiences of shaming by parents during childhood appeared more important than experiences of physical abuse for the development of an abusive personality in adult male batterers.

Childhood exposure to sibling or partner abuse also has been associated with an increased risk in adulthood for child abuse and partner abuse (Alksnis and Taylor, 1994; Kropp et al., 1995; Rosenbaum and O'Leary, 1981; Saunders, 1995). This association reportedly is modest; a finding that is consistent with Widom's (1989) results indicating that only about 30 percent of children physically abused subsequently abused their own children.

Dutton and Hart (1992a) found that men tended to perpetrate, as adults, the same type of abuse they experienced as children. Most studies, however, have not differentiated between specific forms of violence and have instead typically looked at child maltreatment as a general factor.

Egeland (1993) reported that results of the longitudinal study he and his colleagues conducted of high-risk parents and their children, which included psychologically unavailable parents, revealed a 40 percent rate of child maltreatment across generations. Egeland noted that children establish patterns of relating early and develop models of relationships from their early relationship experiences. He concluded, "The violence per se is not passed on from one generation to the next; rather, the ongoing theme of the caregiving relationship is transmitted" (p. 206).

Although the effects of child maltreatment can be severe and lasting, they do vary from case to case, depending on a number of different variables. Research has shown that the frequency and severity of the abusive acts contribute to the negative impact of abuse, as do a variety of other family and environmental variables (Kendall-Tackett et al., 1993). However, other factors, such the child's coping abilities (O'Keefe, 1994; Wolfe, 1987), or the availability of a supportive caregiver (Egeland, 1988), can mitigate the impact of maltreatment.

Furthermore, when conducting child maltreatment risk assessments it is important to remember that self-reports of exposure to violence in childhood may be distorted in either direction. Perpetrators of abuse may overreport being victimized during childhood (Hindman as cited in Murphy and Smith, 1996). In contrast, Della Femina and colleagues (1990) have suggested that offenders also may underreport abusive incidents. Alksnis and Taylor (1994) reported that, as adults, batterers with a childhood history of violence were more likely to idealize their violent parent or rationalize his or her behavior. They noted this finding is consistent with the attachment literature pertaining to abusive mothers who were victimized as children, yet idealized their past.

Socialization Experiences Outside the Home

Exposure to Nonfamily Violence During Childhood

The effects of childhood abuse by a nonfamily member are likely to vary and depend upon factors such as the frequency and severity of the abuse, the child's coping skills, and the reactions and support of others. When the assailant is a stranger, issues involving a betrayal of trust by someone formerly trusted are not involved. However, other issues, such as experiencing the world as unpredictable and violent, may be more prominent.

A review (Lowry et al., 1995) of research pertaining to violent adolescents identified peer pressure to conform to group norms that promote the use of violence, along with violent gang involvement, as influencing factors. The importance of other contributing risk factors such as coming from violent families and communities, access to weapons, and other variables were also noted.

The literature describing the effects of exposure to media violence (Comstock, 1992; Lowry et al., 1995) strongly suggests a positive association between the exposure to nonfamilial and, in this case, impersonal violence and aggressive, antisocial behavior. Such an association, however, does not imply causality because it is unclear whether children who watch excessive violence tend to become violent or whether aggressive children tend to be drawn to violent entertainment. Regardless of the direction of influence, the presence of violent media exposure may signal increased risk in a given case.

Social Competence

Wolfe (1987) defined social competence as the ability "to apply interpersonal skills to meet the demands of the situation and provide positive outcomes for the actors involved" (p. 37). Inadequate or insufficient social competence can be seen in problems in school, work, and interpersonal relationships.

Educational and Academic Functioning

Educational disadvantage and reading deficits have been associated with child maltreatment (Azar, 1989; Brown et al., 1998) and juvenile sex offending (Graves as cited in Weinrott, 1996). Wolfner and Gelles (1993) found a curvilinear relationship between educational level and injurious or potentially injurious acts toward children. Subjects with at least some high school education demonstrated the highest rates of abusive behavior. Higher rates of truancy have been found among juvenile sex offenders who have recidivated (Schram et al., 1991) and dropping out of school early has been associated with partner abuse (Magdol et al., 1998).

Vocational Functioning

Financial and recent employment problems, unemployment, job insecurity, poor work histories, work-related frustration and stress, relationship difficulties with co-workers and bosses, and job terminations have been associated with child maltreatment (Fryer and Miyoshi, 1996; Grayson, 1995; Wolfe, 1987). Parents whose parental rights have been terminated have been described as having difficulty finding or maintaining employment (Schetky et al., 1979). Conversely, relatively stable employment histories have been associated with few acts of interpersonal violence (Webster et al., 1994).

Interpersonal and Relational

Interpersonal relationships and social networks provide people with opportunities to meet their felt needs for affiliation and may provide important emotional and practical supports to help people stabilize and manage their lives at times of stress. Deficits in interpersonal functioning can interfere with an individual's ability to perceive, establish, maintain, and utilize available social supports at times of need.

Deficits in interpersonal functioning may be reflected in attachment problems during childhood. Attachment problems in childhood have been associated with the intergenerational transmission of child maltreatment (Zuravin et al., 1996), juvenile antisocial and adult criminal behavior (Marshall et al., 1993), partner violence (Magdol et al., 1998), and sexual violence (Seidman et al., 1994).

Interpersonal deficits may be expressed in a variety of ways but when severe may be seen through high levels of interpersonal conflict or social isolation. Deficits in interpersonal functioning include problems in familial relationships such as marital, parent-child, or sibling relationships as well as extrafamilial relationships such as peer and work relationships. Problems also may be apparent in dating experiences, nonmarital intimate relationships, and prior marriages.

Furthermore, relationship problems, the lack of adequate social skills, and problems with intimacy have been described as risk factors for juvenile sex offenders (Becker, 1998; Fehrenbach et al., 1986; Friedrich, 1990; Miner and Crimmins, 1995) as well as juvenile delinquents in general (Weinrott, 1996). Similar deficits have been identified in the adult sexual offender literature (Lisak and Ivan, 1995; Pithers et al., 1987; Seidman et al., 1994). Inappropriate age associations can be related to social immaturity as well as pedophilia (Knight, 1992). Never being married is a risk marker for sex offense recidivism (Hanson and Bussière, 1998) and interpersonal violence (Webster et al., 1994).

Relationship instability and intimate violence, including marital or date rape, are obvious areas of concern (Alksnis and Taylor, 1994; Campbell, 1995). Issues such as chronic interpersonal conflict and recent relationship problems have been associated with child neglect (Wolfe, 1985), partner abuse (Kropp et al., 1995), and interpersonal violence (Webster et al., 1995). Parents whose parental rights have been terminated also have been described as experiencing social and interpersonal difficulties, as exemplified by unstable marriages, frequent change of residence, and isolation (Schetky et al., 1979).

In contrast to the relationship between social isolation and impaired interpersonal functioning, social relationships, networks, and services that provide parents with positive support have been associated with adequate parenting and more attachment security in children (Crittenden, 1985b). Supportive interpersonal relationships are considered very important for helping people positively and effectively manage the effects of life stress and problems (Milner and Dopke, 1997). For example, social support has been cited as a key variable in differentiating mothers who broke the cycle of maltreatment from those who did not. In a twelve-year prospective study, Egeland (1988) found that social support during childhood, for example, by a caring foster parent or relative, a positive therapeutic relationship, or a long-term, stable, and intact relationship with a boyfriend or husband differentiated mothers who broke the cycle of abuse.

Lifestyle Impulsivity and Irresponsibility

By definition, characteristics such as lifestyle impulsivity and irresponsibility are inconsistent with social competence. In fact, lifestyle impulsivity and irresponsibility have been identified as being among some of the most prominent factors for increased risk for sexual violence and general violence (Hare, 1991; Prentky and Knight, 1986). Similarly, Brown and colleagues (1998) found maternal sociopathy, defined as experiencing problems with the police or drugs and alcohol, was associated with child physical abuse, sexual abuse, and neglect; paternal sociopathy was associated with child neglect. Marker and colleagues (1999) found parental antisocial behaviors associated with their children having been sexually molested.

Functioning As a Parent

Attachment Histories

Negative maternal attitudes regarding pregnancies, such as when the pregnancy was unplanned or unwanted, have been associated with increased rates of various types of child maltreatment (Brown et al., 1998; Gray et al., 1979; Altemeier et al., 1982; Zuravin and Starr, 1991). This finding may reflect a lack of bonding during pregnancy as may occur during unplanned pregnancies. Early separations from the mother also have been associated with physical abuse and neglect (Brown et al., 1998) and may reflect attachment difficulties.

Similarly, there is an association between nonbiological parents and an increased risk of physical and, especially, sexual abuse (Brown et al., 1998; Milner, 1995; Sedlack and Broadhurst, 1996). This association could be related to nonbiological parents missing the early interactions that may promote the formation of healthy child-parent bonds and inhibit incestuous behavior (Araji and Finkelhor, 1985).

Parents' relationship histories with children can reveal important information about the acceptance of parental responsibilities (Hare, 1991) and the ability to appropriately care for children. Circumstances and patterns of interactions that can disrupt the process of attachment between parent and child have been associated with maltreatment and abuse (Belsky, 1993; Gray et al., 1979; Grayson, 1995; Pianta et al., 1989) and partner violence (Dutton et al., 1995) and have been related to attachment difficulties in infants (Crittenden, 1985a; Youngblade and Belsky, 1989).

Communication and Interactions

Parental sensitivity has been described as involving a parent's ability to provide consistent, contingent, and appropriate responses to an infant or child's cues and signals (Wolfe, 1991). Although parental sensitivity is associated with optimal parenting, parental insensitivity has been related to child maltreatment as well as to cognitive deficits and attachment difficulties in children (Wolfe, 1991).

Research findings (Erickson and Egeland, 2002; Milner and Dopke, 1997; Wolfe, 1987) have indicated that maltreating parents tend to engage in fewer behaviors that stimulate and facilitate the child's sensory, motor, intellectual, and emotional development. They appear to communicate with their children less, provide fewer simple commands and reasoning, fewer positive responses, less contingent praise for appropriate behavior, less verbal and nonverbal instruction, and engage in fewer interactions with their children than nonabusive parents (Brown et al., 1998; Kolko, 2002; Milner and Dopke, 1997; Wolfe, 1991). The interactions that do occur are characterized by a relative absence of positive interactions such as mutual engagement, positive emotional responsiveness, affectionate touch, playful interactions, and mutual pleasure (Azar and Wolfe, 1998; Crittenden, 1996; Grayson, 1995; Milner and Dopke, 1997) and higher rates of commands, directives, and corrections (Diaz et al., 1991). Research also has shown that maltreating parents may behave inconsistently in the ways they respond to their children (Milner and Dopke, 1997).

The reduced frequency of interactions and especially of positive interactions and increased rates of aversive behaviors such as threats and yelling appear to distinguish maltreating parents from non-maltreating parents (Wolfe, 1985) and occur at much greater frequencies than physically abusive acts (Wolfe, 1987). Increased rates of power-assertive and negative parenting interactions have been observed as well (Milner and Dopke, 1997; Oldershaw et al., 1986). In response to their children's perceived transgressions, abusive parents "tend to *reciprocate* the child's aversive behavior rather than attempt to decrease or punish such behavior in an effective manner, thus serving to maintain the coercive exchanges so often found among this population" (Wolfe, 1987, p. 80). However, as Wolfe also observed, other distressed families, apparently without abusive histories, also may have high rates of aversive exchanges and more negative than positive interactions.

Coercive and antagonistic patterns of communication such as yelling, shouting, criticizing, and threatening may be abusive in and of themselves. Actual incidents of physical violence typically occur relatively infrequently (Wolfe, 1987). Yet, aversive and hostile interactions may signal an increased risk for other forms of child maltreatment, including partner violence (Kolko, 2002; McGee et al., 1995; Ney et al., 1994).

Abusive parents also have been found to respond negatively to their children's prosocial behavior. Frodi and Lamb (1980) found that, in addition to experiencing greater negative physiological arousal and aversion to infant cries than nonabusive parents, in contrast to nonabusive parents, they also had negative physiological arousal and emotions in response to infant smiles.

Discipline

Although some maltreating parents have child-rearing skill deficits (Azar, 1989), most possess both developmental information and the ability to articulate appropriate approaches to child rearing (Crittenden, 1996). In stressful situations, however, they appear to have difficulty applying appropriate child management strategies (Crittenden, 1996).

The disciplinary behaviors of maltreating parents reflect less flexibility in understanding children's behavior and greater difficulty generating appropriate child management strategies than controls. For example, punishments may appear to occur randomly, independent of specific child behaviors, suggesting the parent is having difficulty perceiving information or is failing to integrate it (Milner and McCanne, 1991; Milner, 1993), which may contribute to increased difficulties gaining compliance in parent-child interactions (Oldershaw et al., 1986).

Disciplinary approaches tend to involve fewer positive, validating, and affirming comments and increased denigrating and shaming responses (Wolfe, 1991). Interventions frequently are disproportionate, inconsistent, and unpredictable (Wolfe, 1991). Disciplinary techniques tend to reflect an overreliance on authoritarian, power assertion, and punitive approaches, as well as passivity and neglectful avoidance (Belsky, 1993; Milner and Chilamkurti, 1991; Wolfe, 1991), rather than a range of appropriate and effective responses (Milner and Dopke, 1997; Wolfe, 1985, 1987, 1991). An excessive emphasis on achievement, control, and morality has been found in families engaging in severe physical abuse (Barnett et al., 1994).

Maltreating parents tend to express satisfaction with their preferred disciplinary style (Chilamkurti and Milner, 1993; Milner and Dopke, 1997; Wolfe, 1991). A willingness to limit corporal punishment and utilize noncoercive discipline techniques has been associated with increased positive treatment outcomes (Wolfe, 1991). Some maltreating parents, however, have been found to misapply newly learned child management skills such as by using time-out procedures in excessive ways (Azar, 1989).

Supervision and Protection

In addition to failing to provide for a child's physical safety and adequate nutrition, failure to adequately supervise or select appropriate child care providers can be a form of neglect (Barnett et al., 1994; Sedlack and Broadhurst, 1996). Neglectful behavior may be identified when the parent fails to protect the child from accidental or intentional harm on multiple occasions and situations. Inadequate supervision and protection may increase the child's vulnerability to abuse from others. Inadequate supervision also is related to increased rates of juvenile delinquency and future violent behavior (Klassen and O'Connor, 1994). Commitment to protecting the child may be exemplified by the parent's appropriate belief regarding the importance of disclosure of abuse (Iwaniec, 1995).

History of Violent Behavior

A history of violent behavior is an important risk factor for maltreatment. The violence may be intrafamilial or extrafamilial. Targets of violent behavior may include intimates such as children, partners, parents, siblings, and friends, or nonintimates such as acquaintances and strangers. Other forms of "impersonal" criminal aggression, such as armed robbery and the destruction of property, also indicate a history of violence.

Intrafamily Violence

An important historical factor is whether the person has a history of performing family violence. For example, although reports vary concerning how often men who physically assault their wives also physically abuse their children, these forms of family violence co-occur. Jaffe and colleagues (1990) reported one-third, Saunders (1995) found about one-half, and Bowker and colleagues (1988) found as many as 70 percent of men who assault their wives also physically abuse their children. Bowker and colleagues also found more frequent and severe wife abuse was associated with more severe child abuse.

Furthermore, research suggests that women who are abused by their partners are above average in physically abusing their children, although the primary risk to children is from abusive fathers (Saunders, 1995). Children frequently observe partner abuse and, as already noted, this in and of itself can negatively affect them (Alksnis and Taylor, 1994; Edleson, 1999a; Jaffe et al., 1992; Kolbo et al., 1996; O'Keefe, 1994; Miller-Perrin and Perrin, 1999). In addition, higher levels of violence in parent-child dyads have been found to co-occur with higher levels of violence in sibling relationships (Graham-Bermann et al., 1994).

History of Extrafamilial Violence

Studies also vary concerning the frequency with which men who physically abuse their partners also are violent outside the family. In a study that investigated the occurrence of violence toward wives and nonfamily members in a large nationally representative survey involving 2,291 males, Kandel-Englander (1992) found that only 10 percent of the men in the sample were violent toward nonfamily members as well as their wives. In contrast, in a study by Dutton and Hart (1992b), using a criminal offender population, the researchers found 79 percent of the men who had committed some form of family violence also committed some form of stranger or nonfamily violence. It may be that men who are violent toward nonfamily members are more likely to be criminally prosecuted and incarcerated than those who are abusive only within their families (Alksnis and Taylor, 1994). Or, perhaps, perpetrators of extrafamilial violence have higher rates of family violence.

Characteristics of Prior Violence and Maltreatment That Enhance Risk

Age at Onset

Individuals in younger age categories have an increased risk of violence. Being a young or teenage parent has been associated with child maltreatment (Brown et al., 1998; Fryer and Miyoshi, 1996). Miller (1984), however, found that teen mothers were only slightly overrepresented among maltreating parents and that the mothers who were in their early twenties and early thirties were overrepresented in the comparison general population. Mothers over forty-five years were underrepresented. Associations between youthful parenting and maltreatment have been found to dissipate when socioeconomic status is controlled (Mrazek, 1993).

Younger ages have been associated with adult sexual violence (Berliner et al., 1995), partner abuse (Saunders, 1995), and interpersonal violence (Webster et al., 1994, 1995). In addition, younger ages have been associated with treatment dropout rates for maltreating teenage parents (Danoff et al., 1994; Hansen and Warner, 1994) and partner abuse perpetrators (Saunders, 1995).

Number of Prior Episodes

The past is the best predictor of interpersonal violence (Klassen and O'Connor, 1994; Mossman, 1994; Webster et al., 1995; Webster et al., 1994). Previous acts of abuse or violence have been found to be a risk factor for child maltreatment (Grayson, 1995), multiple referrals for child abuse and neglect (English et al., 1999; Marshall and English, 1999), and partner violence (Kropp et al., 1995; Saunders, 1995). Prior incidents of abuse also have been associated with sexual offending (Berliner et al., 1995; Firestone et al., 1999; Hanson and Bussière, 1998; Prentky et al., 1997). Although Hanson and Bussière's (1996) meta-analysis found younger ages associated with sexual recidivism, they noted much variability in the age findings. They concluded that, in regards to sexual recidivism, the relationship between age and sexual recidivism might not be completely linear. In particular, they noted that further research is needed to determine whether sexual recidivism peaks at different ages such as in the twenties for rapists and in the thirties and fifties for child molesters.

Duration of Pattern

Longer-term patterns can be associated with increased risk of recidivism. Antisocial behavior during childhood and adolescence has been related to child maltreatment (Egeland et al., 1991). In addition, significant numbers of adult sexual offenders began their abusive behavior before the age of eighteen years old (Murphy and Smith, 1996).

Klassen and O'Connor (1994) reviewed literature indicating that the rehearsal of violent behavior during adolescence may be a critical factor for the development of adult violence. In fact, these authors asserted that the data suggest the earlier this rehearsal begins, the more likely that the violent behavior will persist into adulthood. For example, they noted that juvenile records are predictive of adult violence in adult psychiatric patients.

Saunders (1995) noted partner abuse frequently does not desist when the relationship ends. He reported that studies (Ganley and Harris, 1978; Pagelow, 1981) have found significant numbers of men who abused their previous partners also abused their new partners. In addition, men who previously abused their partners frequently continued to harass and abuse them after their separations (Epstein and Marder as cited in Saunders; Kelso and Personette as cited in Saunders; Saunders and Size as cited in Saunders, 1995).

Frequency and Escalation

Increasing frequencies or escalating rates of violent behaviors have been associated with life-threatening violence in partner abuse (Saunders, 1995). Boer and colleagues (1997) noted that although empirical support associating the escalation in frequency or severity of violence and risk of sexual offenses has been lacking, anecdotal evidence has provided some support for this association and professionals consider it to be important. Boer and colleagues suggested that such factors are probable risk factors because they reflect other risk factors that have been associated with risk, such as sexual deviation and attitudes supportive of or condoning sexual violence.

Number of Victims

Higher numbers of victims are associated with increased risk. For example, the number of victims has been associated with increased sexual violence (Barbaree and Marshall, 1988; Chaffin, 1994) and partner abuse (Saunders, 1995). In addition, having multiple victims within the family has been associated with multiple referrals for child abuse and neglect (Marshall and English, 1999).

Type of Violent Behaviors

Certain types of violent behaviors are associated with higher rates of relapse. For example, in contrast to incest offenders, who tend to exhibit lower recidivism rates, nonfamilial molesters and rapists appear to have high recidivism rates (Hanson and Bussière, 1998; Marshall and Barbaree, 1990).

Criminal Versatility

Multisituational aggression and a varied pattern of criminal actions are associated with increased risk. Criminal versatility and multisituational aggressive behavior have been found to be risk factors for child abuse and neglect (Wolfe and Wekerle, 1993) and partner abuse (Campbell, 1995; Saunders, 1995).

Sexual assault has been associated with increased rates of partner assault (Campbell, 1995; Saunders, 1995). Campbell and Alford (1989) found that batterers who performed marital rape have higher recidivism rates. Criminal arrest records have been associated with repeated partner abuse (Saunders, 1995).

Nonsexual violent and nonviolent criminal behavior is correlated with repeated sexual violence by adult sex offenders (Chaffin, 1994; Hanson and Bussière, 1998) and with repeat offending by juvenile sexual offenders (Kahn and Chambers, 1991; Miner et al., 1997; Rasmussen, 1999; Schram et al., 1991; Sipe et al., 1998; Smith and Monastersky, 1986). Demonstrating nonviolent criminal as well as violent criminal behavior also is associated with higher rates of interpersonal violence (Webster et al., 1994). The presence of a criminal history has been associated with treatment dropout rates in child maltreating parents (Butler et al., 1994) and partner abusers (Saunders, 1995).

Threatened or Actual Use of a Weapon

Threatening or using a weapon has been associated with an increased risk of partner abuse (Campbell, 1995). Boer and colleagues (1997) reported that research identifying the use of weapons as a risk factor has been lacking, but professionals consider it to be important. They suggested that this is a probable risk factor because it may reflect sexual deviance, possibly sexual sadism, and attitudes that support or condone sexual violence.

Threats of Injury or Death

Threatening injury or death has been associated with partner abuse (Campbell, 1995; Saunders, 1995) as well as treatment dropout in partner abusers (Saunders, 1995). Boer and colleagues (1997) reported that research identifying such threats as a risk factor has been lacking, but professionals consider them to be important. These authors included the category of threats of injury or death with the category of threatened or actual use of a weapon and, as noted earlier, suggested these factors may reflect sexual deviance, possibly sexual sadism, and attitudes that support or condone sexual violence.

Severity and Physical Injury

Performing sexual intercourse during a sexual offense has been found to be a risk factor for repeated sexual violence (Barbaree and Marshall, 1988). In addition, the use of force during a sex offense has been positively associated with sexual recidivism (Barbaree and Marshall, 1988).

Repeated partner abuse and life-threatening partner assaults have been related to the severity of abuse and sadism during previous assaults (Campbell, 1995). Severe partner abuse also has been associated with severe child abuse and poor treatment outcomes (Saunders, 1995). In contrast, victim injury has been negatively correlated with general interpersonal violent recidivism (Webster et al., 1994). Victim injury, however, may be unreliable as a risk factor because it can be associated with situational factors such as the availability of a weapon.

Victim Gender

The association between the gender of the victim and sexual recidivism is unresolved. There appears to be much support for the position that pedophiles with male victims have higher rates of recidivism (Hanson and Bussière, 1998; Marshall and Barbaree, 1990; Quinsey,

Lalumière, et al., 1995). However, other studies have found that males diagnosed with opposite-sex pedophilia had a higher average number of victims than those diagnosed with same-sex pedophilia (62.4 as compared with 30.6) (Abel et al., 1981). Other studies have found no significant differences in the incidence of previous sexual offenses between opposite-sex pedophiles and same-sex pedophiles (Langevin et al., 1985) or in the recidivism rates of child molesters who had abused male versus female victims (Prentky et al., 1997). Complicating the picture still further, others (Abel et al., 1988; Marques, 1995 as cited in Prentky et al., 1997) have found higher re-offense rates for offenders who victimized both boys and girls.

Precipitating Behaviors and Motivations

Nonsexually motivated sexual offenses, for example, sexual offenses that have a strong anger motivation, were found to result in more victim harm and also were more likely to be impulsive than offenses primarily motivated by sexual gratification (Barbaree et al., 1994). Evidence of active ideation, fantasy, or offense planning has been associated with an increased risk of sexual violence (Pithers et al., 1987).

Consequences and Interventions

The need for legal interventions also may be a risk marker. Protection petition court appearances and substitute care have been described as risk factors for serious maltreatment (Murphy et al., 1992). Conversely, the fear of arrest has been associated with reduced rates of partner abuse (Saunders, 1995).

Adjustment problems on conditional release, such as probation or parole, also have been related to interpersonal violence in general (Webster et al., 1995; Webster et al., 1994). Institutional adjustment and management problems have been associated with repeated interpersonal violence (Webster et al., 1994). Conversely, however, positive behavior within an institution may not be informative (Webster et al., 1994).

Biological Factors

Various biological and neuropsychological factors have been associated with sexual violence (Langevin and Watson, 1996) and aggressive and violent behavior (Volavka, 1995). These factors include hormonal, neurotransmitter, electrophysiology, and brain dysfunction. Congenital and genetic factors also may be involved (Raine et al., 1990; Volavka, 1995). Research in this area is limited, however. For example, Quinsey and Lalumière (1996) observed that research findings have not revealed an association between hormonal levels and specific sexual activities or interests.

Complicating this area of study is the possibility that biological and social factors may interact. For example, birth complications and maternal rejection have been associated with violent nonsexual and sexual offenses (Raine et al., 1997). A review of the literature pertaining to the relationship of neurobiology and violence is beyond the scope of this guide.

PERSONAL OR DISPOSITIONAL FACTORS

This area involves a wide range of personal factors concerning cognitive, emotional, personality, and behavioral functioning.

Cognitive Functioning

Level of Intellectual Functioning

Correlational studies have linked lower intellectual functioning with physical child abuse (Milner and McCanne, 1991) and sexual violence (Barbaree and Marshall, 1988). By itself, mental retardation with intelligence quotients below 60 has been associated with neglect. Mental retardation has also been associated with increased risk of neglect when found in combination with other stress factors such as an absence of adequate social support (e.g., financial aid and familial assistance), more than one child, or medical or psychological problems, including a partner's emotional or physical problems (Tymchuk, 1992).

These findings are consistent with other research results that have found low intellectual functioning to be correlated with criminal and violent behavior. It should be noted, however, that this association has not always been supported in the literature (Klassen and O'Connor, 1994) and the specific contribution of low intellectual functioning to abusive or criminal behavior is still unclear.

Volavka (1995) noted that low intelligence, especially low verbal intelligence, contributes to cognitive styles that result in impulsive, uncontrolled responding, without considering future consequences. Volavka also pointed out that low intellectual functioning is related to academic failure during childhood and such failures can reduce the child's attachment to school, thereby interfering with prosocial socialization. Thus, as others (Klassen and O'Connor, 1994) have noted, lower intellectual functioning, like other cognitive deficits, may be a predisposing or contributing factor that, especially when combined with other risk factors, increases the likelihood of maltreating and criminal behavior.

Low intellectual functioning also is related to treatment amenability. For example, Tymchuk (1992) found that many mothers with mild mental retardation could acquire adequate parenting skills and learn to recognize when their skills were not adequate for the health care of their children. For a substantial number of mothers involved, however, many of their treatment gains were quickly lost once treatment was discontinued. Furthermore, when mental retardation is complicated by personality disorders, treatment outcomes are worsened (Gabinet, 1983; Jones, 1987).

It is important to note that, as Melton and colleagues (1997) pointed out, most parents with mental retardation are only mildly retarded and they often are capable of maintaining employment and living independently under normal circumstances. As these authors also noted, mental retardation is strongly correlated with social class and many of the deficits evidenced by parents with mental retardation may, therefore, be confounded with issues of low socioeconomic status and problematic levels of social support (Azar et al., 1995).

In view of these findings, a determination regarding parenting ability should not rest solely on a diagnosis of mental retardation. As can be seen in the following section, increased risk is related to specific skill deficits that may be more common in mentally retarded individuals, for example, deficits in problem solving, abstract thought, or cognitive flexibility, rather than the mere diagnosis of mental retardation itself. To the extent that mental retardation signals these deficits, it may be a marker of risk, but this would be true in a given case only if the assumed skill deficits were in fact present in ways which were related to issues of maltreatment in the particular case.

Other Cognitive and Neurological Deficits

Problem Solving. Problem solving and decision making difficulties, particularly in child-related situations, have been identified in parents who maltreat their children (Azar et al., 1984; Egeland et al., 1991; Milner and Dopke, 1997). Poor judgment and difficulty planning ahead have been found in parents whose parental rights have been terminated (Schetky et al., 1979).

Mosher and Righthand (1995) have proposed that successful problem solving in child care situations will involve the ability to do the following:

1. Accurately identify problems
2. Conceptualize alternative problem-solving strategies
3. Assess the strengths and weaknesses of various options
4. Implement strategies
5. Evaluate the strategies' success
6. Self-correct, as needed, by selecting strategies that promote long-term goals versus short-term relief

Abstract reasoning and cognitive flexibility. Deficits in abstract reasoning and cognitive flexibility contribute to difficulties in understanding children's behavior and generating appropriate child management strategies (Milner, 1993; Milner and McCanne, 1991). Abusive parents engage in less induction and reasoning when they discipline (Chilamkurti and Milner, 1993). Conversely, Milner and Dopke (1997) cited an unpublished controlled study (Nayak and Milner, 1995) that found that the risk of physical abuse decreased as conceptual ability, cognitive flexibility, and problem solving increased.

Cognitive deficits and impairment also have been associated with aggressive behavior in general (Klassen and O'Connor, 1994; Volavka, 1995). Individuals with cognitive deficits who become abusive and violent may have difficulty anticipating the negative consequences of violent behavior, may not be able to resolve difficulties verbally, or may not have the resources necessary for complex problem solving (Volavka, 1995).

Perceptual accuracy. Parents who maltreat their children tend to have distorted perceptions and attributions of others (Egeland et al., 1991; Milner and Dopke, 1997; Reiss Miller and Azar, 1996). As a group, "Maltreating parents tend to think in global, all-or-nothing terms rather than see the shades of gray that more realistically capture human behavior" (Erickson and Egeland, 2002, p. 13). These individuals typically show limited insight, lower levels of emotional awareness, and diminished capacity to take the perspective of others (Dougher, 1995; Dutton, 1995; Egeland et al., 1991). In addition, neglectful parents may be so withdrawn, emotionally unavailable, and/or depressed that they may fail to perceive their children's cues and signals (Crittenden, 1993).

Such perceptual inaccuracy can interfere with the parents' awareness of their children's needs. These inaccuracies can result in distortions of the child's behaviors, strengths, weaknesses, and special needs. For example, parents who are evaluated as presenting a high risk for perpetrating child physical abuse have been found to make fewer attributions of competence in their children (Diaz et al., 1991). Maltreating parents frequently are described as having trouble seeing things from a child's perspective, as well as understanding and appreciating the relationship between child behavior and developmental level, situations, and contextual factors (Erickson and Egeland, 2002).

Physically abusive parents frequently perceive their children's behavior as more stressful (Wolfe, 1991) and more negative than others do (Reiss Miller and Azar, 1996). In addition, high-risk parents tend to view their children's personal and conventional transgressions as more wrong than low-risk parents, and perceive power assertive disciplinary techniques as more effective (Chilamkurti and Milner, 1993).

Maltreating parents also may have difficulty differentiating their own needs from those of their children (Hess et al., 1992; Wolfe and Wekerle, 1993). For example, parents whose parental rights had been terminated tended to place their own needs before those of their children's and viewed their children as existing to satisfy their needs (Schetky et al., 1979). Similarly, a substantial number of disrupted family reunifications (69 percent) involved parents placing children at risk in order to meet their own needs (Hess et al., 1992). Although this practice may be due to the parents' difficulty in accurately perceiving the children's needs, it also can result when the parent has little regard for what is in the children's best interests.

Problems in accurately perceiving others also are found in partner abusers (Dutton, 1995; Saunders, 1995) and sex offenders (Dougher, 1995; Lisak and Ivan, 1995; Murphy and Smith, 1996; Seidman et al., 1994). Deficits in their perceptual accuracy of social and emotional cues have been observed.

Attributional styles. The cognitive and attributional styles of maltreating individuals tend to be more negative than those of non-abusive people (Egeland et al., 1991; Reiss Miller and Azar, 1996). This includes their attributions about themselves, others in general, and their children in particular.

Milner and Dopke (1997) suggest that maltreating parents differ from controls in the amount of internal responsibility and hostile intent (Reiss Miller and Azar, 1996) that they attribute to their children for their behaviors. For example, in one sample, abusive parents were found to minimize their personal responsibility for negative parent-child interaction as well as minimize their children's role in positive interactions (Bradley and Peters, 1991).

Physically abusive parents also report that their children engage in more negative behaviors, particularly in marginal situations, suggesting preexisting attributions and beliefs may bias their evaluations of their children's behaviors (Milner and Dopke, 1997). Even in the face of mitigating information, high-risk parents are less likely to alter their negative child-directed attributions (Milner and Dopke, 1997).

The general propensity of high-risk parents to attribute hostile intent to others (Reiss Miller and Azar, 1996) can interfere with their ability to access social supports when they are available.

Attitudes and beliefs. Various attitudes, values, beliefs, and rationalizations are associated with child maltreatment (Egeland et al., 1991). Attitudes and beliefs about parenting, including the importance attached to the parenting role (Iwaniec, 1995), can be important risk factors. For example, verbal and behavioral indicators reflecting ambivalence about assuming the parental role and initiating reunification have been associated with failed reunification efforts (Hess and Folaron, 1991). Likewise, attitudes involving fears of spoiling the child and beliefs in the value of punishment have been associated with abusive parental behavior (Grayson, 1995). Conversely, positive attitudes toward service and treatment providers and expectations for treatment success have been associated with positive treatment outcomes in maltreating families (Grayson, 1995).

Sex offenders also frequently are described as showing a range of cognitive distortions and thinking errors (Dougher, 1995; Griffiths et al., 1989; Pithers et al., 1987; Murphy and Smith, 1996; Quinsey and Lalumière, 1996). Attitudes that support or condone sexual offenses (Ageton, 1983; Blumenthal et al., 1999) and negative attitudes toward women have been associated with sexual offending (Lisak and Ivan, 1995). In addition, sex role stereotypes, patriarchal attitudes, and attitudes that support partner abuse have been related to men perpetrating partner violence (Kropp et al., 1995; Saunders, 1995).

Expectations of Child Behavior

Although research findings have been mixed (Milner and Dopke, 1997), some studies have found that physically abusive parents have greater unrealistic expectations of their children as compared to other parents (e.g., Azar et al., 1984). Milner and Dopke (1997), however, have found that abusive parents had lower expectations than comparison groups. In either case, such expectations appear unrelated to the child's needs or abilities (Wolfe and Wekerle, 1993).

Research findings also suggest that abusive parents may have developmentally inappropriate expectations of children's needs, especially pertaining to complex behavioral interactions (Milner and Dopke, 1997). They also may have lower expectations of child's compliance after discipline for serious transgressions and higher expectations of child compliance following minor transgressions (Milner and Dopke, 1997). Furthermore, their expectations regarding everyday behavior typically are more rigid (Milner and Dopke, 1997).

Emotional Functioning

Research has demonstrated a positive relationship between emotional arousal, negative mood states, and maltreating behaviors (Crittenden, 1996; Goodman and Brumley, 1990; Milner and Dopke, 1997). Milner (1993) argued that evidence from the social information processing literature suggests that emotional arousal and mood states can influence social information processing activities such as perceptual accuracy.

Furthermore, when experiences are stored in memory, they can be laden with affective charges and recollections of emotional memories can be facilitated by similar mood states (Bower, 1981). As a result, current stresses or conflicts may be exacerbated if, for example, the parent selectively attends to negative cues or previous experiences. Current circumstances may stimulate memories of previous aversive experiences that, in turn, may act to intensify the parent's emotional arousal and reaction. Wolfe (1987) suggested that these mood and memory associations might lead to a cycle of maltreatment. The arousal of angry and dysphoric emotions may interfere with rational problem solving. Harsh discipline, based on emotion and reflex, may be justified as necessary or blamed on the child. Subsequently, this rationale may be remembered and used to justify future instances of harsh discipline or maltreatment.

Emotional instability has been identified by Pianta and colleagues (1989) as the best predictor for differentiating parents who maltreated their children from those who provided good care. Maltreating parents have been described as easily irritated and annoyed, showing low frustration and stress tolerances, and having difficulty in expressing and controlling their anger (Egeland et al., 1991; Milner and Dopke, 1997; Wolfe and Wekerle, 1993). More specifically, physically abusive parents have been found to have a lower threshold for child misbehavior and to be more physiologically reactive to stressful child-related stimuli than comparison groups (Friedrich et al., 1985; Kolko, 2002; Milner and Dopke, 1997). Hyperarousal and increased psychophysiological responsiveness as evidenced by physical tension and increased pulse rate and respiration in response to child-related behavior have been associated with physical abuse (Milner, 1993; Milner and Dopke, 1997). Such hyperresponsiveness also can contribute to more general patterns of information processing difficulties, problem-solving difficulties, and impulsive behaviors that interfere with relationships and parenting (Kolko, 2002; Milner, 1993).

Neglectful parents also have been found to have greater physiological reactions to stressful child-rearing situations (Friedrich et al., 1985). Similar to physically abusive mothers, and unlike controls, neglectful patients had more difficulty habituating to the sound of a baby's cry than controls. The neglectful parents also were most aroused by the sound of a noxious, but not child-related sound, again suggesting difficulty in habituating and relaxing in the presence of such aversive stimuli.

Habitual patterns of stress can result in states of chronic emotional arousal, overgeneralization, and deficient regulation. For example, a parent might think, "No matter what I do he won't listen" (Wolfe, 1987, p. 66). Conversely, habitual stress and arousal also may lead to the types of detachment, distancing, and joylessness that have been observed in maltreating parents during parent-child interactions (Milner, 1993; Oldershaw et al., 1986).

Few studies have investigated the relationship between emotional regulation and sex offending. Pithers and colleagues (1987) noted that, contrary to theories purporting that many sexual acts were impulsive, their analyses of the precursors to sexual assault revealed that more than half of the offenders in their study appeared emotionally over-controlled and inhibited. These individuals tended to avoid expressing angry emotions when such feelings were first aroused. Instead, they brooded about the incident over time, and their anger intensified. Their sexual assaults were considered a delayed emotional expression of their anger and rage. This group, however, contrasts with other types of sexual aggressors, such as the "pervasively angry" rapist described by Knight and Prentky (1990). The global and undifferentiated anger of these sex offenders permeates all aspects of their lives.

Sexual Functioning

Sexual preoccupation with children (Prentky et al., 1997) and sexual preference for children as measured by phallometric methods (Hanson and Bussière, 1998) are risk factors for sexual recidivism. Similarly, "deviant sexual preference," a more general category including rape as well as molestation, also has also been associated with sexual recidivism in adults (Hanson and Bussière, 1998) as well as juveniles (Weinrott, 1996) whether measured by self-report or phallometric methods.

Sexually deviant fantasies are presumed to have an important role in the etiology and maintenance of sex offending; however, empirical research that supports this view remains limited (Langevin et al., 1998). Langevin and his colleagues studied a sample of adult male sex offenders who had admitted their offenses in comparison to a community-based control group and a nonviolent offender group with no known sexual offenses. Their findings indicated that reports of deviant fantasies by all of the groups were low, that only a third of the sex offenders reported deviant sexual fantasies, and that the groups could not be reliably differentiated on the basis of their sexual fantasies. The authors suggest that sex offenders, like other individuals, may vary from each other. They noted that some sex offenders may have limited or even no sexual fantasies of any kind whereas for others sexual fantasies may be more important. For example, as Langevin and colleagues (1998) noted, perpetrators of serial sexual homicides have been found to have higher rates of sadistic or sexually violent fantasies than perpetrators of single sexual homicides (Prentky et al., 1989). Prentky and colleagues suggested that such deviant sexual fantasies might be a way serial offenders rehearse their offenses. Fortunately, as Langevin and colleagues pointed out, sexual sadists comprise a small portion of sexual offenders and, as Prentky and colleagues noted, a relatively small, but unknown, number of individuals who have sadistic sexual fantasies attempt to act them out.

Personality Functioning

Early research efforts regarding child maltreatment emphasized the role of parental personality characteristics and psychopathology. Subsequently, research found that severe parental psychopathology is not typically present (Wolfe, 1987). Most studies, however, have found that parental "emotional problems" are associated with child maltreatment and certain personality factors have been associated with child maltreatment (Milner and Dopke, 1997). These include the following.

Attachment Style

Mothers with insecure adult attachment styles (ambivalent or avoidant) have been found to be significantly more at risk for perpetrating child abuse (Moncher, 1996). Related factors included lower trust and confidence in relationships, frustration with partners, and clinging to partners. Ambivalence within relationships and jealousy and fears of abandonment were significant, but less strongly correlated. Anxious relationships between higher-risk mothers and their partners have been described in other research as well (Crittenden, 1996).

In addition, hypotheses relating poor parent-child attachment to later histories of juvenile and adult sexual offending have received some research support (Marshall et al., 1993; Seidman et al., 1994). Rapists, for example, have been found to have less motivation for intimacy than controls (Lisak and Ivan, 1995).

Attachment difficulties, particularly a fearful attachment style, also have been identified in men who engage in partner violence (Dutton et al., 1995).

Apathy

Apathy has been associated with neglect. Polansky and colleagues (1981) described an "apathy-futility syndrome" among neglecting mothers who presented as passive, withdrawn, and lacking in emotional expressions. They appeared to have the conviction that nothing was worth doing, lacked competence in many life skills, and had interpersonal relationships characterized by desperate clinging, superficiality, an absence of pleasure, and intense loneliness. In addition, these mothers tended to express anger passive-aggressively, were verbally nonexpressive, and had significant problem-solving difficulties.

Domineering, Controlling Interpersonal Style

Rigid, domineering, controlling interpersonal styles have been associated with child physical abuse (Milner, 1994; Wekerle and Wolfe, 1993) as well as partner violence (Saunders, 1995).

Emotional Immaturity

Immaturity, in general, has been specifically associated with parental neglect (Crittenden, 1996). When operationalized as the parent expecting the child to care for the parent, parental emotional immaturity also has been associated with broader forms of child maltreatment (Wolfe and Wekerle, 1993). Mothers who abused their children and who engaged in, but did not benefit from, treatment, have been described as infantile, immature, and inadequate (Gabinet, 1983).

Empathy

Empathy is considered an inhibitor of general aggression because it is believed to promote behaviors incompatible with aggression, such as helping behaviors (Milner and Dopke, 1997). Empathy deficits have been associated with specific forms of violence such as physical abuse (Milner and Dopke, 1997), child maltreatment (Grayson, 1995; Wolfe, 1991), and sexual violence (Lisak and Ivan, 1995; Marshall and Maric, 1996). Empathy deficits also have been identified in parents whose parental rights have been terminated (Schetky et al., 1979).

Empathy deficits may not consistently occur across contextual and temporal situations, however (Milner, 1998; Pithers, 1999). For example, Pithers found that sex offenders experienced a contextual empathy deficit when they experienced emotions that were precursors to abuse.

External Locus of Control

Parents who engage in physical child abuse have been described as having an external locus of control that involves powerful others and chance factors (Bradley and Peters, 1991; Brown et al., 1998; Milner and Chilamkurti, 1991; Milner, 1994). In contrast, neglectful parents have been described as perceiving themselves as well as others as powerless. For these parents, experiences frequently are explained as the result of "luck and fate" rather than self-efficacy (Crittenden, 1996).

Impulsivity

Impulsivity has been associated with parents who engage in child abuse and neglect (Friedrich et al., 1985; Nelson et al., 1993; Wolfe and Wekerle, 1993), as well as with parents whose parental rights have been terminated (Schetky et al., 1979).

Passive-Dependency

Some maltreating parents have been described as passive and dependent in their interpersonal relationships (Grayson, 1995; Hess et al., 1992). A study by Friedrich and colleagues (1985) reported test results that suggested neglectful and abusive parents were significantly more dependent, helpless, and passive than low-income, non-maltreating controls.

Pervasive Anger and Hostility

Pervasive or chronic hostility has been associated with physical child abuse (Kolko, 2002; Friedrich et al., 1985; Milner and Dopke, 1997) and neglect (Brown et al., 1998; Friedrich et al., 1985). Hostility may be expressed through irritability, annoyance, anger, and aggression as well as passive aggression, such as refusing to talk about difficulties. Maltreating parents have been described as frequently expressing covert hostility, for example, by covering their hostility with falsely pleasant behavior (Crittenden, 1996).

Pervasive anger has also been associated with a subgroup of rapists (Knight and Prentky, 1990). Pervasive anger and hostility has been inconsistently found in men who engage in partner assaults. The rates of assault, however, increase when anger exists and is focused specifically on the marital relationship (Saunders, 1995).

Self-Concept and Self-Esteem

With few exceptions, studies have found low self-esteem is directly or indirectly associated with child maltreatment (Christensen et al., 1994; Grayson, 1995; Milner and Dopke, 1997; Schetky et al., 1979). For example, studies (as cited in Milner and Dopke, 1997) have found low self-esteem is associated with increased negative perceptions of children and reduced ability to adequately manage family stress. More specifically, Melton and colleagues (1997) reported that a low sense of competence as a parent, along with emotions appropriate to that self-perception (such as depression) might be the most validated characteristic of maltreating parents.

Conversely, narcissistically inflated levels of self-esteem, combined with situations or circumstances that threaten the individual's highly favorable self-perception, have been associated with higher rates of violence (Baumeister et al., 1996). Consequently, inflated self-esteem may be a risk factor for child maltreatment.

Personality Disorders

As noted above, severe parental psychopathology is not commonly a factor in cases of child abuse and neglect (Wolfe, 1987). However, severe personality disorders and personality dysfunction have been associated with parents maltreating their children (Egeland et al., 1991; Murphy et al., 1992). For example, parents with antisocial personality disorders have been found to be 25.7 times more likely to engage in child neglect (Swanson et al., 1994).

Personality disorders and personality dysfunction also have been correlated with sexual violence (Chaffin, 1994; Pithers et al., 1987; Scalora, 1989) and interpersonal violence (Limandri and Seridan 1995; Webster et al., 1995; Webster et al., 1994). For example, research has shown that narcissism is especially associated with partner violence (Saunders, 1995). A personality disorder combined with anger, impulsivity, narcissism, or behavioral instability also is associated with increased risk for criminal behavior, including violent behavior (Kropp et al., 1995).

Psychopathy

High rates of interpersonal violence, sexual offending, and partner abuse have been associated with psychopathy (Firestone et al., 1999; Forth, 1995; Hare, 1996; Hill et al., 1996; Rice and Harris, 1997; Saunders, 1995; Serin et al., 1994; Webster et al., 1995; Webster et al., 1994).

Perceived Stress

Higher levels of perceived life stress have been associated with child maltreatment (Milner, 1993; Pianta et al., 1989). Maltreatment has been related to parents feeling overwhelmed and unable to cope (Egeland et al., 1991). Controlled studies have not, however, found actual differences in the levels of real life stress experienced by maltreating parents as compared with nonmaltreating parents (Milner, 1995; Milner and Dopke, 1997; Wolfe, 1991).

The importance of perceived life stress also is seen in cases of interpersonal violence (Webster et al., 1995). Research findings pertaining to the relationship between perceived life stress and partner abuse, however, have been inconsistent (Saunders, 1995).

To account for the critical role perceived life stresses may have in the development of child maltreatment, Hillson and Kuiper (1994) have developed a "stress and coping" model of child maltreatment. As part of this model, the authors suggest that child neglect may be associated with parents responding to stress with behavioral disengagement, mental disengagement, the suppression of competing activities, and dysfunctional social support seeking. In contrast, child abusers may rely on venting emotions. Nonmaltreating parents may differ from both groups by utilizing active planning and coping, restraint coping (e.g., not acting while enraged), functional social support seeking, and positive reinterpretation. The authors pointed out, however, that all parents may use strategies from each category, and that the coping strategies of neglectful and abusive parents, in particular, may overlap.

Coping Responses, Internal Resources, and Motivation for Change

Just as risk factors can increase the risk of child maltreatment, other factors may reduce or mitigate the risk. In addition to contextual factors and situational variables, such factors include positive coping responses and internal resources and influences.

Coping Skills

Hillson and Kuiper (1994) have noted that the stress and coping literature describe a number of characteristics associated with effective stress management. These include personal resources such as high levels of ego strength and self-esteem, a sense of coherence, a belief in mastery, cognitive flexibility and complexity, good analytic abilities, knowledge, and interpersonal skills. Coping skills may include a variety of positive emotional and problem solving abilities such as rational problem solving, relaxation skills, recreational activities, and so forth. These characteristics and coping skills contrast with the types of immediate, ineffective, and maladaptive approaches such as emotional venting, interpersonal disengagement, or the dereliction of responsibilities that often are seen in cases of child maltreatment (Grayson, 1995; Hillson and Kuiper, 1994; Wolfe, 1987).

Ability to Perceive and Access Social Supports

Social supports can provide important functions such as "emotional and material support, knowledge information, appraisal support (information pertinent to self-evaluation), and companionship" (DePanfilis, 1999). However, certain psychological characteristics such as suspicion, feeling threatened, social alienation, negative attribution toward others and antisocial sentiments may interfere with a person's ability to perceive social supports as accessible. Likewise, these factors also may interfere with an individual's ability to access supports even if they are perceived as available (Azar, 1997).

Motivation and Readiness for Change

When assessing risk and the prognosis for positive behavioral changes, the question is not simply whether the parent can make necessary and appropriate changes to adequately meet their child's basic developmental needs, but whether the parent can become able to meet each child's needs within a time frame consistent with the child's developmental requirements. To answer this question evaluators must assess how able, ready, and motivated the parent is to make necessary changes. The parents' past and current responses to interventions may provide important information about their prognosis for positive behavioral change.

The role of motivation in the process of behavioral change has recently received increased attention. The importance of assessing an individual's motivation for change has been applied to child maltreatment interventions (Gelles, 1996), sex offender treatment (Kear-Colwell and Pollock, 1997), and partner abuse interventions (Dutton, 1996; Gondolf, 1987).

Current models of motivation conceptualize the readiness for change as involving five stages (Prochaska et al., 1992). These include the following:

1. Precontemplation
2. Contemplation
3. Preparation
4. Action
5. Maintenance

In the precontemplation stage, the individual does not perceive the need for change. In fact, the person may not even perceive there is a problem. As an individual moves from the precontemplation stage to the contemplation stage there is recognition of the need to change, but ambivalence about committing to the required course of action. People frequently become stuck in the contemplation stage for extended periods (Prochaska et al., 1992). The third stage, preparation, involves formulating plans and taking minor steps toward change. In contrast, an individual in the action stage is fully involved in plan implementation. The final stage, maintenance, is reflected by relapse prevention activities.

Although sequential, the authors of this model (Prochaska et al., 1992) are careful to note that individuals may regress as well as make progress across these stages as they grapple with any problem. For example, if an individual is unable to implement their plan at the action phase, he or she may regress to the preparation stage to reformulate the plan (positive response) or regress to the contemplation stage, where there is ambivalence about the necessity for change (negative response).

The Stages of Change Model is consistent with theories and research that has shown associations between issues such as resistance to treatment and negative attitudes toward interventions and child maltreatment, sexual violence, and partner abuse recidivism. For example, Dewhurst and Nielsen (1997) proposed that sex offenders in the precontemplation and contemplation stages frequently present with varying levels of denial, dissimulation, minimization, and cognitive distortions. People in the precontemplation stage may not even perceive that there is a problem, and when this is so, they are at an increased risk for dropping out of treatment (Jones, 1987). In addition, future expectations and plans (preparation) have been included in risk assessments of sexual violence (Boer et al., 1997) and interpersonal violence in general (Webster et al., 1994). Specific behavioral steps (action), such as keeping appointments, have been associated with improved treatment outcome in maltreating parents (Grayson, 1995). Likewise, relapse prevention has been described in the sexual violence literature as an approach that may help individuals maintain treatment gains and behavioral control and thereby avoid reoffending (Hall et al., 1993; Pithers, 1987).

CLINICAL OR SYMPTOM FACTORS

Most of the people who are evaluated for child maltreatment, sexual abuse, or partner violence are not mentally ill. Research does not support conclusions about a person's parenting abilities or propensity for violence based solely upon a mental illness or diagnostic category (Melton et al., 1997). In fact, Melton and colleagues reported that research findings have shown that some mothers with severe mental illness appear to have been able to adequately care for their babies even during an acute psychotic episode. This finding is consistent with other research, which compared patients discharged from a psychiatric hospital with community controls. Steadman and colleagues (1998) found that the violence prevalence rates among both patients and control groups who are without symptoms of substance abuse did not differ significantly. Rates of violence increased for both groups when substance abuse symptoms were present.

The risk impact of psychiatric diagnoses, including mental illness and other disorders, may be best understood when evaluated in combination with other risk factors (e.g., Limandri and Seridan, 1995). It is the combination of disorders and deficits such as substance abuse, cognitive deficits, limited positive social supports, and treatment compliance problems, along with a history of abusive or neglectful behavior that may increase the risk of child maltreatment and violence. Thus, when diagnoses are considered in concert with other information, such as the history of maltreatment, parenting skills, and motivation for change, they may be very relevant indeed.

As Dyer (1999) noted, the *Diagnostic and Statistical Manual of Mental Disorders,* Fourth Edition (DSM-IV), provides specific behavioral and interpersonal descriptions of characteristics associated with various disorders, many of which are very relevant for child maltreatment risk assessments.

> If the examinee meets the criteria for a specific personality disorder or presents traits and features of more than one disorder, the DSM-IV can be a useful bridge from the clinical data underlying the diagnosis to citation of specific defects in the individual's parenting capacity that would signal unfitness. (p. 111)

Specific Clinical Symptoms

Although mental illness, as a general category, is too broad to be of much use in assessing the risk of maltreatment, specific symptoms have been noted in the literature as increasing the risk of violent behavior. These include hallucinations and delusions, conceptual disorganization, threatening mannerisms, posturing, grandiosity, suspiciousness, and agitation (Limandri and Seridan, 1995; Link and Stueve, 1994).

Murphy and colleagues (1992) found that psychotic illnesses, along with character disorders, frequently were present when child maltreatment cases returned to court. Furthermore, parental psychosis with delusions involving their children have been found in parents who reabused their children in spite of treatment (Jones, 1987).

A study of child fatalities (Margolin, 1990) related to parental neglect did not find caregiver psychosis or clinical depression to be a common factor. In fatality cases involving physical abuse, however, four of the forty-eight deaths were described as related to command hallucinations or delusions that focused on the child and another four deaths were associated with the parent's suicide or suicide attempt.

Suicidal ideation or behaviors have been associated with partner violence (Campbell, 1995) and homicide and violence in general (Kropp et al., 1995). More general patterns of violent thoughts or behaviors also may imply increased risk (Campbell, 1995; Kropp et al., 1995).

Milner and Dopke's (1997) review of the empirical literature indicated that although severe psychopathology may be associated with very severe forms of child assault in individual cases, serious psychopathology typically is not a factor in cases involving physical abuse. They noted, however, that parental emotional problems are an issue and reported, as noted earlier, in one study (Pianta et al., 1989) emotional instability was found to be the best predictor for differentiating parents who maltreated their children from those who provided good care.

A range of dysphoric and unpleasant emotions has been associated with child maltreatment (Pianta et al., 1989; Egeland et al., 1991; Friedrich et al., 1985; Milner and Dopke, 1997; Wolfe, 1991). These include feeling anxious, sad, unhappy, depressed, hopeless, distressed, lonely, annoyed, irritable, angry, hostile, aggressive, and suspicious.

Assessment may be difficult because hostile interchanges sometimes may be present during seemingly pleasant interactions such as smiles and playful or affectionate behaviors (Crittenden, 1996). Neglect is more commonly associated with depression (Crittenden, 1996).

Such negative emotions also have been associated with sexual assault (Pithers et al., 1987; Seidman et al., 1994) and partner abuse (Saunders, 1995). Generalized anger and anger toward women have both been associated with sexual violence (Pithers et al., 1997). Hostility toward women and marital anger has been associated with partner abuse (Saunders, 1995). Depressed moods have been associated with partner abuse, but only inconsistently so (Saunders, 1995). Parental characteristics such as being depressed or having an antisocial history also have been related to in-session resistance at all phases of treatment (Patterson and Chamberlain, 1994).

Substance Abuse

Substance abuse, as with other psychiatric diagnoses and disorders, should not be considered in isolation when evaluating a parent's ability to parent in nonmaltreating ways. The interaction between the substance abuse and other historical, dispositional, symptom, and situational factors must be assessed.

Substance abuse has been found to co-vary with child maltreatment (Yoast and McIntyre, 1991), increased rates of multiple referrals for child maltreatment (English et al., 1999), sexual offending (Firestone et al., 1999), and partner violence (Magdol et al., 1998). However, research has not demonstrated a causal relationship (Yoast and McIntyre, 1991) and as Azar et al. (1998) have noted, an individual's use of substances may vary over time, and research identifying factors associated with such variations is limited.

In a large epidemiological study investigating mental health disorders, substance abuse, and child abuse, Kelleher and colleagues (1994) found that parents' lifetime history of alcohol abuse and their physical abuse or neglect of their children were strongly associated. Even after controlling for other known risk factors such as depressive disorders, number of persons in the household, antisocial personality disorders, and social supports, substance abuse or dependence continued to be strongly associated with child abuse and neglect. Parents with an alcohol or drug disorder were 2.7 times more likely to have reported abusive behavior toward children, and 4.2 times more likely to have reported neglectful behavior toward children than matched control subjects.

Empirical research into the effects of parental substance abuse, especially alcohol abuse, on children is limited (Melton et al., 1997). Substance abuse and particularly drug abuse has been related, however, to increased social isolation, social mobility, parental psychological unavailability, and physical neglect (Melton et al., 1997). Substance abuse also has been associated with increased rates of children reentering foster care (Hess et al., 1992).

Substance abuse, especially in combination with other psychiatric diagnoses (including personality disorders), has been correlated with higher rates of interpersonal violence in general (Swanson, 1994; Steadman et al., 1998). Substance abuse also has been associated with severe partner abuse and victim injury (Saunders, 1995). Limandri and Seridan (1995) noted, however, that other factors, such as expectations and beliefs regarding substance abuse and the frequency of substance abusing behavior, as contrasted with the occurrence of violent behavior, must be considered before causal relationships can be suggested.

CURRENT SITUATION AND CONTEXTUAL FACTORS

Current situation and contextual factors are those circumstances that increase or mitigate risk at the present time. These factors focus on what the child would experience if he or she were in the home today. Some of these variables may be static and others may be transient.

Victim Factors

Victim access is an obviously important situational variable (Monahan, 1981). Inadequate supervision of children can increase their exposure to hazardous situations and potential perpetrators over time.

Victim Age

Findings from the *Third National Incidence Study of Child Abuse and Neglect* (NIS-3) (Sedlack and Broadhurst, 1996) revealed that older children, usually defined as over two or over five years old, have higher rates of maltreatment. Rates appear to increase in the middle childhood years (six to eleven years). Other studies (Egley, 1991; Wolfner and Gelles, 1993) also have shown that physical child abuse and neglect peak among preschool- and middle childhood-aged children as compared with infants, toddlers, and teenagers. Rates of sexual abuse of children appear to increase after age three years (Sedlack and Broadhurst, 1996). It is the youngest children, however, who appear at greatest risk of death from child maltreatment. This vulnerability of very young children is demonstrated by findings that only 10 percent of children who have died as a result of child maltreatment were older than four years old (U.S. Department of Health and Human Services Administration for Children and Families, 1995).

Interpretations of these age differences include the possibility that the maltreatment of preschool children is underdetected because it is less observable by people outside the family situations (Belsky, 1993; Sedlack and Broadhurst, 1996). As Seagull (1997) observed, "Younger children are potentially less safe . . . because they are physically more fragile and developmentally less able to protect themselves by leaving a dangerous situation or asking for help" (p. 154). In contrast, as noted by Sedlack and Broadhurst, teenagers may be more able to avoid maltreatment by removing themselves from the situation.

Regardless of the variability in victim age, early onset has been associated with multiple referrals for child abuse and neglect (Marshall and English, 1999). Furthermore, the physical and developmental vulnerability of infants and preschoolers to maltreatment must not be overlooked. Young children spend more time with their parents and are more physically and psychologically dependent upon them (Belsky, 1993). Because of their small size and physical limitations, they are especially vulnerable to adult physical force.

Furthermore, young children have increased difficulty regulating their emotions. The sometimes defiant self-assertions of these children as well as the oftentimes clinging and dependent behaviors that they exhibit may serve to stimulate aggressive responses in some parents.

Victim Gender

Findings from the NIS-3 (Sedlack and Broadhurst, 1996) revealed that girls are sexually abused three times more often than boys. Boys, however, have a greater risk of serious injury, as well as emotional and physical neglect, than girls do (Sedlack and Broadhurst, 1996; Wolfner and Gelles, 1993).

Research findings suggest that most incest offenders do not evidence sexual preferences for children or have gender-specific arousal patterns (Quinsey and Lalumière, 1996). Their arousal patterns, as measured by phallometric assessment, typically show age and gender preferences similar to non–sex-offender control groups.

Victim Characteristics

Parent-child interaction theories (Azar, 1989; Miller-Perrin and Perrin, 1999) suggest that certain factors, such as whether a child is temperamentally more difficult than most children, is developmentally delayed, or is simply very young and needy, may interact with parental behavior problems and deficits. Such factors may aggravate anger control difficulties, negative attribution biases, and poor parenting skills.

Azar and colleagues (1998) noted that

> The literature on children with disabilities . . . suggests that disabled children make demands at multiple levels: the immediate family (e.g., greater financial and time resources), the extended family (e.g., respite care resources), the physical environment (e.g., a home with handicap access), and the community (e.g., access to a clinic that best serves their needs). Over time these needs may change and the parent needs to be able to recognize when they change and how to adjust his or her behavior accordingly or find assistance from those who can. (p. 94)

Seagull (1997) noted that "developmentally disabled children are less able to protect themselves . . . and . . . can be more difficult to care for, thus placing them at increased risk" (p. 154). There is some empirical support for this concern. For example, Marshall and English (1999) found higher rates of multiple referrals for child abuse and neglect among parents of children with developmental delays. Also, Ammerman and his colleagues (1994) found that 61 percent of children and adolescents with developmental disabilities experienced some form of severe maltreatment by a caregiver in their lifetime.

However, research into the possible relationship between a child's medical, intellectual, and developmental characteristics and his or her risk of maltreatment have produced mixed findings (Belsky, 1993; Kolko, 1996a). Perhaps, as Belsky noted,

> If, as is now widely acknowledged, maltreatment is a transactional byproduct of processes taking place between parent and child in a family and community context, then studies . . . that examine "main effects" of child characteristics are likely to underestimate the interactive role that factors like prematurity and handicap play in the etiological equation. (pp. 419-420)

Social and Economic Factors

Economic Poverty

Studies (Bath and Haapala, 1993; Brown et al., 1998; Crittenden, 1996; Fryer and Miyoshi, 1996; Sedlack and Broadhurst, 1996; Wolfner and Gelles, 1993) have consistently shown that rates of child maltreatment, especially child neglect, are correlated with economic poverty. For example, the NIS-3 (Sedlack and Broadhurst, 1996) found families with income levels below $15,000 were twenty-two times more likely to evidence some form of child maltreatment than families that had income levels above $30,000.

Although economic poverty is a risk factor for child maltreatment, and partner abuse as well (Magdol et al., 1998; Saunders, 1995), the relationship is not causal. As with other risk factors, economic disadvantage does not act in isolation and should not be used in isolation to draw conclusions about a specific case. Various problems associated with economic poverty may underlie the correlation between economic poverty and increased risk, and these associated issues may not be present in all cases where there is economic poverty.

Family Structure

Single-parent status has been associated with neglect (Bath and Haapala, 1993; Brown et al., 1998; Fryer and Miyoshi, 1996) and physical abuse (Brown et al., 1998; Milner, 1995). Findings from the NIS-3 indicated that in comparison to children living in two-parent households, children of single parents had a 77 percent increased risk of being harmed by physical abuse and an 87 percent increased risk of being harmed by physical neglect (Sedlack and Broadhurst, 1996).

Large family size also has been related to child maltreatment and especially to neglect (Brown et al., 1998; Grayson, 1995), physical abuse (Bowker et al., 1988; Milner, 1995), and fatal neglect (Margolin, 1990). Wolfner and Gelles (1993) found a curvilinear relationship between minor and severe violence toward children and number of children in the family, with a peak occurring at four or five children.

As discussed earlier, the presence of a nonbiological parent (Brown et al., 1998; Milner, 1995; Sedlack and Broadhurst, 1996) may increase risk, especially for sexual abuse. Most children who are maltreated, however, are abused or neglected by birth parents (Sedlack and Broadhurst, 1996).

Home Environment

Lack of privacy as well as unsafe and crowded housing has been related to maltreatment (Wolfe, 1987). In addition, fathers who are unemployed and, especially, fathers who are employed part-time, appear to present more risk of abuse than fathers who are employed full-time (Wolfner and Gelles, 1993). These factors may reflect economic disadvantage, opportunity and access to victims, as well as increased stress.

Inadequate household management and environmental hazards also have been associated with child maltreatment (see Grayson, 1995).

Residential Stability

Transience has been related to child maltreatment and treatment compliance (Belsky, 1993; Butler et al., 1994; Fryer and Miyoshi, 1996). In addition, child placement in foster care followed by reunification has been associated with multiple referrals for child maltreatment (Marshall and English, 1999).

Neighborhood Quality

In a study of community factors and child maltreatment, Garbarino and Kostelny (1992) found that, in neighborhoods with higher than predicted maltreatment rates, the "general tone" of visits to this community was depressed. During interviews people had trouble finding anything good to say about their community, tended to know less about available community services, and had fewer formal and informal support systems than did people in communities with lower maltreatment rates. In addition, visits to this community revealed that, "the physical spaces of the programs themselves were dark and depressed, and to a casual visitor the criminal activity was easily spotted" (p. 461).

Child-Parent Dyad and Interactive Factors

A number of child-parent dyad and interactive factors have been associated with an increased risk of child maltreatment. As noted earlier, research has demonstrated that child maltreatment is a significant risk factor for attachment insecurity and associated relationship disturbances (Carlson, 1998; Carlson et al., 1989; Cicchetti et al., 1995; Crittenden, 1988; Lynch and Cicchetti, 1991; Main and Solomon, 1990; Schuengel et al., 1999). Attachment difficulties stemming from interactions between the parent and the child may reflect attachment problems that originate with the parents, the child, or both. Ongoing child and parent attachment difficulties and disorders are likely to further disrupt the parent-child relationship and negatively affect the child.

In addition, parental dissatisfaction with the child (Brown et al., 1998) and unrealistic parental expectations when measured in terms of the child's abilities increase risk (Grayson, 1995). Increases or decreases in real or perceived child behavior problems also can be related to maltreatment. Although child behavior problems never justify maltreatment, a child's behavior may be a stimulus that interacts with abusive or neglectful parenting practices. For example, parental discipline strategies, whether punitive control or noncoercive techniques, tend to be repeated when they are reinforced by the child's compliance or submission (Wolfe, 1987).

For children who are placed in substitute care, changes in functioning associated with different placements and visitation schedules may provide information about the parent-child relationships. Visitation consistency when the child is out of the home may reflect the parent's attachment to the child. Such interpretations should be made with caution, however, because visit inconsistency could result from practical difficulties as well (Azar, 1996).

Child and parent reactions to each other on visits also may provide important information about their relationship, but this data should not be simply taken at face value (Azar et al., 1998). For example, distress after visitation can suggest that the parent-child contact is detrimental for the child, or it may be that the separation is causing the distress (Fahlberg, 1997).

Current Family Functioning and Patterns

In addition to parent-child relationships, current patterns of adult-to-adult and sibling relationships within the family may contribute to risk. For example, ongoing conflict and violence in the parent's intimate relationship (Brown et al., 1998; Hess et al., 1992; Milner, 1995) have been associated with child maltreatment (Fryer and Miyoshi, 1996; McKay, 1994; Milner, 1995; Saunders, 1995; Shipman et al., 1999; Wolfe and Wekerle, 1993). Furthermore, partner violence has been associated with multiple referrals for child maltreatment (Marshall and English, 1999).

Such conflicts and violence also have been related to sexual violence (Campbell and Alford, 1989; Pithers et al., 1987), and repetitive partner abuse (Saunders, 1995). Perceived threats of, or the actual loss of the relationship, has been identified as risk factors for partner violence (Kropp et al., 1995), perhaps especially among individuals most psychologically threatened by perceived or actual abandonments (Holtzworth-Munroe and Stuart, 1994).

Family instability, disorganization, and chaos also have been associated with child maltreatment (Barnett et al., 1994; Crittenden, 1996; Gray et al., 1979; Wolfe, 1985), and extreme disorganization and chaos has been found to be especially characteristic of families where children have been sexually abused (Pianta et al., 1989). Unstable adult relationships frequently are present in cases of child maltreatment, with mothers often being unmarried, divorced, or separated (Crittenden, 1996).

Other family factors have been associated with child maltreatment and family violence. These include fewer overall frequencies of family interactions and greater frequencies of negative interactions (Crittenden, 1996; Milner and Dopke, 1997; Wolfe, 1987). As noted earlier, hostile interchanges may be present during seemingly pleasant behaviors, such as smiles and playful or affectionate behaviors (Crittenden, 1996). As this author states, assessment of these issues may be especially complicated because individuals may vary their interactional style across persons and situations.

Social Supports

Social support can enhance parental competence in many ways. For example, in addition to providing practical assistance such as child care, supportive individuals can assist parents by modeling effective and positive parenting techniques. Drawing on the research of Cutrona (1984) concerning predictors of postpartum depression, Wolfe (1987) noted that supportive individuals also may help enhance parental competence by "facilitating problem solving, increasing access to accurate information about children and parenting practices, fostering opportunities for positive reinforcement, and affirming worth in the parenting role" (p. 38).

Comprehensive and frequent supports of sufficient duration that occur within the home and are provided by specially trained staff have been found to reduce abuse rates in mentally retarded parents (Tymchuk, 1992). Comprehensive programs that provide such support and supervision also have aided physically abusive, nonretarded parents (Wolfe and Wekerle, 1993).

In contrast, social isolation and other deficiencies in social support, including the type and quality of available social support, have been associated with neglect (Crittenden, 1985b), physical abuse (Milner and Dopke, 1997), and combined types of child maltreatment (Bishop and Leadbeater, 1999; Crittenden, 1985b; Wolfe and Wekerle, 1993). A lack of adequate social supports also has been associated with juvenile sex offending (Fehrenbach et al., 1986; Miner and Crimmins, 1995; Visard et al., 1995), and more general patterns of interpersonal violence (Webster et al., 1995).

The effects of social support, of course, can depend upon the nature of the associations. It does not appear that research efforts have addressed this particular issue as it pertains to parents who have maltreated their children. Criminal, deviant, and subcultural identifications have been strongly associated with juvenile delinquency and violence (Lowry et al., 1995; Hawkins et al., 1998). The relationship between antisocial peers and criminal recidivism has been shown to be paramount in adult offenders as well (Gendreau et al., 1996). In addition, associations with other sex offenders may be a possible risk factor for sexual reoffending (Hanson and Scott, 1996).

Such findings are not limited to negative peer group affiliations. For example, Knight and Tripodi (1996) found that as youths committed more crimes, their parental attachments increased. The authors believed this finding could be related to the fact that 70 percent of the parents in this study had been incarcerated and, as such, they have their criminality in common.

Cultural as well as environmental barriers can interfere with the parents' ability to access positive social supports (Azar et al., 1995). For example, a variety of difficulties may interfere with client participation in treatment programs. These difficulties may include cost, transportation problems, lack of child care, waiting lists, or excessive geographic distance (Miller and Rollnick, 1991). Other problems may involve shyness or safety concerns, language barriers, or cultural attitudes about discussing one's personal problems (Azar et al., 1995; Miller and Rollnick, 1991; Preciado and Henry, 1997).

FINAL REMARKS

As noted earlier in this chapter, risk assessment involves identifying factors that research has found may increase or mitigate risk. One objective of risk assessment is to identify the risk of future child maltreatment that individuals or families may present. Another objective is to design interventions for effectively managing risk. The next chapter addresses the very important issue of formulating risk management strategies.

Chapter 4

Formulating Risk Management Strategies

INTRODUCTION

The probability of child maltreatment is increased when risk factors exceed protective factors and stresses outnumber supports (Cicchetti and Lynch, 1993). Successful intervention in cases of child maltreatment involves shifting this equation by reducing stress and increasing protective factors (Schellenbach, 1998).

The challenge in developing effective risk management strategies, however, is to translate these broader conceptual factors into specific targets that are amenable to intervention. A variety of factors make this challenge a complex and difficult task. First among these factors is the multisystemic nature of child maltreatment. In his ecological model of child maltreatment, Belsky (1980) noted that multiple factors influence the occurrence of child maltreatment. These include individual (ontogenic) factors, family (microsystemic) factors, community (exosystemic) factors, and cultural (macrosystemic) factors. To be most effective, interventions may be required at each of these levels and, consequently, involve multiple, coordinated targets and providers who are sensitive to class and cultural differences.

It is important that interventions designed to interrupt maltreating behaviors and to facilitate parental sensitivity to the child's developmental stage identify parental strengths as well as vulnerabilities; the child's strengths, needs, and special needs, if present; as well as environmental stresses and supports. Effective interventions also require sensitivity to the developmental needs of children and parents as individuals and also as parent-child dyads, family members, and members of their communities whose patterns of interactions change over time (Cicchetti and Rizley, 1981).

Many factors can complicate interventions and interfere with effective treatment. Hansen and colleagues (1998) report that such factors include

> (1) The presence of multiple stressors and limited financial, personal, and social resources within the family for coping with stressors, (2) the often coercive nature of the referral and the possibility that participation in services may be involuntary or under duress, (3) the fact that abusive behavior cannot be readily observed, and (4) the need for many different interventions to treat several target areas. (p. 133)

Other factors that confound treatment efforts include situations where maltreating parents have cognitive limitations and may not be able to benefit from verbal and insight-oriented therapies (Wolfe, 1994). Too many interventions, poor timing of interventions, or interventions that are inappropriate to their targets may overwhelm clients, resulting in reduced effectiveness and wasted resources (Crittenden, 1996).

Families who have maltreated their children are a heterogeneous group and, as such, require individualized interventions tailored and timed to maximize their effectiveness (Hansen et al., 1998). As Egeland and colleagues (2000) point out, "The indiscriminate implementation of an intervention program for high-risk parents is doomed to failure unless the program identifies the unique needs and circumstances of each family [and each individual family member] as part of the intervention program" (p. 73).

Effective interventions often require prioritizing. As Egeland and colleagues (2000) observe, parents in high-risk samples frequently "struggle with multiple challenges and barriers in their own lives that need to be addressed before they can devote themselves to improving their relationships" with their children (p. 71). Such challenges may include situational demands and stress, such as the need for food and adequate, safe housing; sleep disturbances; financial difficulties; vocational problems; and medical and mental health problems. Challenges also may involve partner violence, substance abuse, the negative impact of the parent's childhood maltreatment experiences, psychopathology, and the developmental needs of a young parent (Egeland et al., 2000; Wolfe, 1985).

Further complicating attempts to provide interventions that may reduce the potential or actual negative effects of child maltreatment, either by prevention or treatment, is the limited empirical data available on what works (Hansen et al., 1998; Kolko, 1998). "The problem lies partially in the fact that research designs are so incredibly difficult to implement under the circumstances (e.g., heterogeneous population, multiple problems and stressors, multiple etiological and maintaining factors, inability to randomly assign subjects to control or comparison conditions)" (Hansen et al., 1998, p. 134). As a result, existing studies typically are descriptive reports that provide limited information about subjects in the study and typically lack comparison or control groups (Wolfe, 1994). These studies almost exclusively focus on mothers and generally involve small samples. When follow-up studies have been employed, they usually have been of relatively short duration and have not assessed long-term recidivism or the effects of the interventions on child development or the parent-child relationship (Schellenbach, 1998).

The intent of this chapter is to briefly review findings from the treatment outcome literature and highlight interventions and programs that, in spite of the aforementioned methodological problems, research studies suggest may be effective in reducing the risk of child maltreatment or ameliorating the negative effects of past maltreatment. More detailed reviews and compilations of this literature may be found elsewhere (for example, Araji, 1997, and Becker, 1998 [sex offending by children and adolescents]; Becker and Murphy, 1998 [sex offending]; Berliner, 1997 [victims of sex abuse]; DePanfilis, 1996a [child neglect]; Kolko, 1998 [child abuse]; Lutzker, 1998 [child abuse]; Saunders and Williams (1996) and Schellenbach (1998) [child abuse]; Wekerle and Wolfe, 1993; and Wolfe, 1994 [child abuse and neglect]). When considering any treatment intervention, however, the limitations of the existing research should be kept in mind.

TREATMENT OUTCOME LITERATURE: A BRIEF REVIEW

Prior to the mid-1980s, theories about the causes of child maltreatment emphasized personality disturbances in parents and recommended psychodynamic interventions to address these personality issues (Azar, 1997; Grayson, 1995). As noted in Chapter 3, however, an individual's parenting abilities or propensity for violence cannot be predicted solely on the basis of the presence or absence of a psychiatric disorder and diagnosis (Limandri and Seridan, 1995; Melton et al., 1997). In addition, research has not generally supported the utility of psychodynamic interventions with people who have maltreated their children (Videka-Sherman as cited in Wolfe, 1994). Psychodynamic approaches have been described as impractical due to the length of time they require (Azar, 1989), because children cannot afford to wait years for their parents' behavior to change. They also require a level of motivation and psychological sophistication that frequently is not found in parents who engage in child maltreatment (Azar, 1989).

The problem of ineffective interventions is not limited, however, to more traditional psychological approaches. Even interventions specifically designed for maltreating parents have fallen short. For example, intensive family preservation approaches frequently have had disappointing results, particularly when child neglect is an issue (Bath and Haapala, 1993). Cohn and Daro (1987) found that one-third or more of the parents served by intensive family preservation programs continued to maltreat their children while in treatment, and over one-half of the families continued to be considered to present a substantial risk for engaging in maltreatment.

Most studies evaluating the effectiveness of interventions with maltreating parents have focused on cognitive and behavioral approaches. The results of these studies suggest that cognitive-behavioral approaches are most likely to be effective when distinct risk factors are identified and then addressed through specific interventions, such as by enhancing child-rearing skills, anger management strategies, and coping abilities (Wekerle and Wolfe, 1993; Wolfe, 1994). Cognitive-behavioral interventions with children who have been maltreated have demonstrated some encouraging results as well. For example, studies have found improvements in social competence, self-concept, and remediation of developmental delays (Wekerle and Wolfe, 1993; Wolfe, 1994).

In spite of the encouraging findings regarding cognitive-behavioral interventions in child maltreatment cases, such approaches have limitations (Wolfe, 1994). For example, these interventions do not address economic or social factors, nor do they address longstanding mental health problems, such as personality disorders and mental illnesses, when these are present. Wolfe concluded, "Given that a wide range of different problems often must be addressed with each family, cognitive-behavioral services may offer the greatest benefit in conjunction with other types of services" (p. 250). For example, comprehensive and ecobehavioral programs that assume that the causes of child maltreatment are multifaceted and extend beyond individual skill levels or the parent-child relationship (Wolfe, 1994) appear more effective (Cohn, 1979; Cohn and Daro, 1987; Grayson, 1995; Wolfe, 1994).

Research studies suggest that programs spanning from one to three years and providing a personalized approach appeared most successful (Cohn and Daro, 1987). Egeland and colleagues (2000) noted that a longer duration of treatment is associated with more positive outcomes, but he observed that the intensity of treatment may vary and that families may benefit from periodic sessions following the completion of more intensive interventions to reinforce treatment gains.

Not all cases require lengthy treatment. One study found that parenting interventions lasting between six and eighteen months have been considered most successful (Cohn, 1979). Daro and McCurdy (1994), however, caution that although child development knowledge can be transferred to parents relatively quickly (i.e., six to twelve weeks), changing attitudes and strengthening parenting and personal skills often require longer interventions.

PARENTING TRAINING INTERVENTIONS

Research suggests that parent-training programs have shown some success (Azar et al., 1995). Methodological problems, such as short follow-up periods, limit these findings, but research does support the conclusion that some of these interventions are effective with some individuals (Grayson, 1995; Wekerle and Wolfe, 1993).

Parent training interventions typically focus most on increasing the individual parent's skill levels in the areas of positive verbal and nonverbal interactions and providing positive, consistent discipline (Azar, 1989). These interventions focus on behaviors and typically use concrete demonstrations and rehearsal to develop effective parenting skills. Therapeutic strategies may include systematic instruction, modeling, rehearsal, and feedback (Wolfe, 1991). Skill development emphasizes noncoercive discipline techniques involving positive reinforcement, using effective verbal strategies that may increase child compliance with parental commands, and using appropriate affect and voice tone during parent-child interactions. Parents are taught to establish appropriate rules and consequences, design behavioral contracts, and implement anger management techniques in stressful parent-child interactions (Azar, 1989; Wolfe, 1985, 1987). Other necessary skill-building approaches may include developing effective problem solving and planning abilities and interventions that address inadequate coping skills, excessive anger, impulse-control problems through stress, anger, and impulse management strategies (Griffiths et al., 1989; Lutzker et al., 1998; Marshall et al., 2000; Wolfe, 1985, 1991).

Parent training interventions may also work to expand or modify the parent's knowledge base by improving awareness of child development and addressing negative attitudes and cognitive distortions concerning parenting and children. Interpersonal goals may include developing empathetic and clear communications and interactions, correcting patterns of miscommunication, including affective miscommunications (Azar, 1989), and enhancing parent-child attachment (Azar, 1989; Wolfe, 1985).

Offense-specific interventions may also focus on the cognitive components that contribute to maltreatment by addressing cognitive distortions, misattributions, negative attitudes, and mistaken beliefs that frequently characterize these parents (Azar, 1989; Egeland et al., 1991; Milner and Dopke, 1997; Reiss Miller and Azar, 1996) as well as the child victim (Azar, 1997; Berliner, 1997). Individuals who have perpetrated abuse may have cognitive distortions about the impact of the abuse on the child, the family system, other individuals, and themselves. Consequence training may help increase the individual's acknowledgment of the problem, facilitate treatment, and promote relapse prevention (Griffiths et al., 1989).

Skill training objectives for maltreating parents may need to extend beyond individual parenting skills to include the goals of enhancing adult interpersonal relationships and social supports (Egeland et al., 2000; Lutzker et al., 1998; Murphy and Smith, 1996). Helping parents develop healthy attachments to other adults can enhance the parents' empathy for and tolerance of children's needs and feelings, as well as increase their ability to access support from others (Zuravin et al., 1996). Specific interventions in this area may include social skills training, assertiveness and communications training, responsibility training (personal, interactive, social, and moral), facilitating interpersonal problem-solving skills, developing social perspective, and empathy training (Azar, 1989; Griffiths et al., 1989; Lutzker et al., 1998; Wolfe, 1991). Once an individual has developed sufficient social skills, social network interventions such as parent education programs and support groups can decrease social isolation. Furthermore, they may help the parent develop support networks, enable sharing of feelings, increase understanding of parental responsibilities, and become more aware of different and effective approaches to child rearing, as well as promote self-esteem, increase social skills, and improve social competence.

COMPREHENSIVE AND ECOBEHAVIORAL PROGRAMS

Comprehensive and ecobehavioral programs assume that the causes of child maltreatment are multifaceted and extend beyond individual skill levels or the parent-child relationship (Wolfe, 1994). As Berliner (1997) noted, many families for whom child maltreatment is a problem also "suffer from the associated consequences of a myriad of environmental, physical, and psychological conditions, including poverty, illness, substance abuse, and criminality. These families often seem to lurch from crisis to crisis and to be overwhelmed by the exigencies of simply surviving" (p. 163). Comprehensive and ecobehavioral programs typically provide overlapping interventions in a variety of settings such as the home, schools, and the community.

In spite of the limitations in our knowledge base as described above, existing research does suggest that approaches which combine parental intervention with a wider range of other supportive services as supplements to professional and lay services have had increased success (Cohn, 1979; Cohn and Daro, 1987; Grayson, 1995; Wolfe, 1994). Evaluations of these treatment programs also have found that comprehensive packages of services that address both the interpersonal and concrete needs of all family members have been most successful (Cohn and Daro, 1987). For example, intensive group and home-based interventions that provide parental support and instruction in child management and cognitive stimulation have had strong positive effects on parental attitudes and behavior and overall maternal adjustment (Wekerle and Wolfe, 1993).

An example of a comprehensive intervention program includes Project 12-Ways (Lutzker et al., 1998). Project 12-Ways initially targeted twelve areas of interventions. The areas were: parent-child training, stress reduction, basic skill development for children, money management, social support, home safety training, multiple setting behavior management, health and nutrition, problem solving, marital counseling, alcohol abuse referral, and single mother services. Lutzker and his colleagues (1998) have found research support for Project 12-Ways.

> Data from single-case research designs have documented the effectiveness of the ecobehavioral approach to child maltreatment by showing skill development in parent training . . ., stress reduction . . ., marital counseling . . ., home safety assessment and hazard reduction . . ., infant stimulation and health care skills, affect training . . ., home cleanliness, and nutrition. . . . Program evaluation data have consistently shown that when compared to a matched comparison group in the same region, families who receive services from Project 12-Ways are significantly less likely to be reported again for child abuse and neglect up to four years after services. . . . Also, in one evaluation, it was determined that Project 12-Ways families were more severe than comparison families prior to treatment. (p. 241)

Project 12-Ways was successfully replicated with parents who have developmental disabilities and live in an urban setting. It also has been replicated with a large Latino population in an urban California setting. Nurses and caseworkers in these other settings replaced graduate students who provided services at the earlier sites.

In contrast to these positive reports, Kolko (1998) has found that more recent applications of this program have shown variability in outcomes. Some interventions have had positive results, whereas others have shown minimal effects. The reasons for these differences were not clear.

Project SafeCare is an ecobehavioral program that extended the Project 12-Ways program to families with young children (birth to five years old), and parents who had been adjudicated for child abuse or neglect or who were considered to be at high risk for maltreating their children. In contrast to Project 12-Ways, Project SafeCare provides intervention in three core areas: child health care, parent-child interactions (bonding), and home safety and accident prevention. Recent outcome results are encouraging. Gershater-Molko and colleagues (2002) found families who participated in Project SafeCare had significantly lower reports of child maltreatment at a twenty-four-month follow-up than families who participated in family preservation programming. In addition, Kolko (1998) reported, "These curricula are noteworthy for their analysis of content validity based on professional reports, simplified checklists of specific parental behaviors, and use of training routines that promote behavioral competency" (p. 229).

Other comprehensive programs that center on children include Multisystemic Therapy (MST) and Multidimensional Treatment Foster Care (MTFC). MST is an empirically based intervention that has been validated with chronic juvenile delinquents and substance abusing youths (Henggeler et al., 1998). MST confronts antisocial behavior in youths by targeting their "social-ecological context" (e.g., their family, neighborhood, school, and community) (Henggeler et al., 1998, p. vii).

Ten years ago, MST was applied to the area of child abuse and neglect. A comparative analysis of MST with other behavioral parent training programs for abusive parents revealed positive outcomes for MST on comparisons between pre- and posttreatment measures using self-report and observational assessments (Kaufman and Rudy, 1991). This study, however, was limited by methodological difficulties, including its small sample size and the lack of subject follow-up. Further research with this approach in the areas of parental child abuse and neglect appears lacking. MST also is the only approach that has been empirically validated as effective with juvenile sex offenders (Weinrott, 1996), however, again the sample size was small and the comparison treatment did not involve current treatment approaches.

MTFC is another empirically based intervention that has been validated with youths with histories of serious juvenile delinquency (Chamberlain and Reid, 1998). Similar to MST, MTFC is ecologically oriented in that it provides interventions for youths in the community through specialized foster care placements. Also along the lines of MST, MTFC involves multiple treatment modes and targets including individual therapy or skill development, family therapy, and school performance and peer groups. Family interventions include significant training and support for the foster family, as well as interventions with the birth family or other family with whom the youth will live following foster care. Community and peer interventions target risk factors associated with the development of antisocial and delinquent behavior (Chamberlain and Moore, 1998).

Chamberlain and Reid (1998) evaluated the effectiveness of MTFC for youths with chronic and severe histories of juvenile delinquency, including some who had committed sexual offenses. They randomly assigned subjects to traditional community group placements or MTFC. Results indicated that youths in MTFC had significantly fewer criminal referrals and returned home to relatives more often than those in traditional group settings did. Multiple regression analyses showed that assignment to the treatment condition (MTFC) predicted official and self-reported criminality more effectively than well-known predictors did.

Treatment foster care and therapeutic foster care are not new approaches, but services and treatment protocols can vary. The Pressley Ridge Youth Development Extension (PRYDE) is another comprehensive, treatment foster care program with empirical support (Fisher et al., 1999). The interpretations of the PRYDE program's positive findings, however, were limited by the lack of random assignment.

Recently, Fisher and colleagues (1999) observed that treatment foster care programs typically serve only elementary school-age children and adolescents. Recognizing the need for early intervention, as well as the placement of very young children in residential care, they developed an age-appropriate program for preschool children in foster care who had been maltreated. This program is the Oregon Early Intervention Foster Care (OEIFC) and is based upon the empirically validated program for older children. It targets three primary areas for child-focused intervention identified by research as risk factors for future difficulties across multiple domains: behavior problems, emotional regulation, and developmental delays.

The nature of most of the OEIFC treatment components is similar to those used with the older children, but they are designed to be developmentally appropriate (e.g., using stickers as part of a behavioral program rather than a complex point system). A couple of interventions are specific, however, to this population. They include the involvement of an early interventionist who works with the child in various settings (such as home and preschool or day care). In addition, the children participate in a weekly therapeutic playgroup that is scheduled concurrently with the foster parent support and supervision group. OEIFC includes the biological family in treatment interventions through family therapy and parent training. The program provides for a gradual reunification process as well. Fisher and colleagues (1999) noted that initial findings from their pilot program showed improved foster parenting and behavioral and emotional regulation by the children, but further evaluation is required.

In addition to agency-based comprehensive programs that center on children, systems of care and wraparound interventions, which have been designed for children with serious emotional disturbance and their families, may prove useful for reducing the risk and impact of child maltreatment. The core principles of these approaches (Goldman, 1999; Kamradt, 2000; Meyers et al., 1999) appear very positive for engaging individuals, families, and communities in the provision of needed and effective interventions. For example, the principles include providing children with individualized, holistic, culturally competent interventions in or as close to a child's home or community as possible and utilizing varied approaches as indicated by drawing upon a range of professional disciplines and agencies working together in an integrated fashion. The principles and approaches include outcome-focused assessment with objective measures.

When child maltreatment is an issue, however, some of the principles may require some modifications or additional methods to assure child safety and welfare. For example, the principles stress that family members are considered partners in treatment planning, implementation, and outcome. They also have "the lead voice as well as choice in decisions regarding treatment plans for their children" (Meyers et al., 1999, p. 11). Interventions also emphasize the strengths and capabilities of the individuals, family, culture, and community instead of deficits when addressing challenges and problems.

Involving parents who have maltreated their children in interventions and emphasizing their strengths appear to be very important strategies for effecting positive change. However, when parents have maltreated their children, safeguards will be needed to ensure that treatment plans are in their children's best interests and that an emphasis on strengths does not miss risks that may indicate the occurrence or likelihood of further maltreatment.

CHILD-CENTERED SERVICES AND TREATMENT INTERVENTIONS

Assuring child safety is of the utmost importance. This may be accomplished through in-home services and supports or by placing the child or children in an alternative placement. Resolving the immediate circumstances of jeopardy, however, does not necessarily eliminate the effects of maltreatment (Daro and McCurdy, 1994). Developmentally appropriate, specialized treatment interventions may be required.

Chapter 2 reviewed the negative effects of child maltreatment that may be reflected in children's short- and long-term behavioral, emotional, and cognitive adjustment. As indicated in that review, maltreatment may disrupt the development and resolution of stage-salient issues such as affect regulation, the development of attachment, the development of the self-system, peer relationships, and school adjustment. The potential long-term impact of poorly negotiated stage-salient issues may include the following:

1. Affect regulation difficulty progressing to behavioral problems
2. Attachment difficulties that affect self-other differentiation, peer relationships, and the development of intimacy
3. Developmental delays that can interfere with academic performance, social relationships, the development of social competence, and a range of other difficulties

The negative effects of child maltreatment will vary in any given case depending on a variety of factors. As noted in Chapter 2, these factors include the nature and duration of the maltreatment, the child's adjustment, family stability, and the availability of social supports. In some cases the impact of the maltreatment may be so severe as to require hospitalization, such as when an absence of nurturing and emotional neglect contributes to an infant's nonorganic failure-to-thrive (Culbertonson and Willis, 1998).

The effects of maltreatment also depend on the child's stage of development at the time of intervention (Daro and McCurdy, 1994). The type, intensity, and duration of interventions will depend on the individual needs of the child. Interventions need to be "developmentally guided" (Wolfe, 1994, p. 237).

In addition to being tailored to the individual needs of the child, therapeutic services for children who have been maltreated should focus on all aspects of the abusive experiences, including the underlying psychological abuse that accompanies most, if not all, forms of abuse (Daro and McCurdy, 1994). Furthermore, in addition to the research on the impact of child maltreatment, research on risk factors associated with the perpetration of child maltreatment and other forms of violence, as described in Chapter 3, reflect the need for child-focused interventions to also facilitate children's social competence.

In his review of interventions for children who have been maltreated, Wolfe (1994) noted that in spite of methodological limitations, preliminary findings from evaluations of child-focused interventions "seem favorable in meeting some of their interventions needs" (p. 246). Children evidenced reduced levels of aggression and improvements in their self-concept and their social, emotional, and cognitive development. He noted, however, that the studies were limited by primarily focusing on young children. The studies also typically did not evaluate the success of concurrent parental interventions or control for the effects of various types of maltreatment.

Abuse-Focused Interventions

Terms such as abuse- or trauma-specific or abuse- or trauma-focused therapy refer to approaches that organize treatment around the abuse experience (Berliner, 1997). Berliner noted abuse-focused interventions are based on the premises that negative psychosocial effects are associated with abusive experiences and that clearly associating these negative effects with the abusive experiences will enhance treatment outcomes.

Friedrich (1996) pointed to two of the few existing child maltreatment comparative studies as supporting treatment interventions that focus directly on abusive experiences. These studies were Kolko's (1996) research with physically abused children and Deblinger and colleagues' (1996) work with children who had been sexually abused.

Both studies compared those who received interventions that addressed abusive behaviors with those who received standard community care. Friedrich noted that in both instances, results supported "the relative efficacy of a planned intervention in which parental abusive behavior (Kolko, 1996) or the sexual abuse experience (Deblinger et al., 1996) was a focus" (p. 344). He also noted that effective interventions (Berliner and Saunders, 1996; Deblinger et al., 1996) addressing post-traumatic stress disorders and other arousal-based symptoms associated with sexual abuse also involve directly targeting the symptoms associated with the trauma or abuse, for example, symptoms of fear and anxiety.

Multifamily group therapy (MFGT) has been compared with traditional family therapy in the treatment of children who have been maltreated and the parents who were abusive (Meezan and O'Keefe, 1998). Families were randomly assigned to MFGT or the comparison group. Although subjects in both groups improved in some areas after treatment, subjects in the MFGT group had significantly lower child abuse potential and significantly greater social support scores on standard measures. Replication and follow-up studies are needed, but these preliminary findings suggest that MFGT may benefit some of these children and their families.

Day Treatment Programs

Child-focused interventions include therapeutic day treatment programs also known as therapeutic child care (Moore et al., 1998; Wolfe, 1994). Most often, these programs provide services to preschool-age children. They provide individual and group approaches. Interventions generally involve parents, but they may be effective even in the absence of parental involvement (Daro and McCurdy, 1994). Developmental delays such as motor problems, sensory difficulties, language delays, and social and emotional difficulties are primary targets of intervention.

Daro's (1988) review of nineteen demonstration child maltreatment intervention projects revealed that therapeutic daycare services were more effective than other interventions at reducing the likelihood of a child being reabused during or after treatment. Furthermore, in a controlled study (Culp et al., 1987), children involved in a comprehensive therapeutic day treatment program demonstrated more improvements in various areas of development than did children who were not in the program. Another study (Culp et al., 1991) also found developmental gains as well as improvements in the children's self-concept and social acceptance.

The importance of therapeutic child care as an early intervention program also is suggested by a twelve-year follow-up study of children who were maltreated or considered at risk of maltreatment (Moore et al., 1998). Subjects were randomly assigned to an ecological-model therapeutic child care program or to standard community services. Data collection involved multiple informants, including the youth, caregivers, teachers, home observations, as well as school and court records. At early adolescence, youths who received therapeutic child care appeared significantly less likely to engage in violent delinquency or display clinical levels of depression and anger. At follow-up, the homes of treated youths were significantly more supportive of adaptive child development and the youths' levels of functioning also appeared more positive than the functioning of the nontreated youths. In addition, children who had received standard community treatment entered the juvenile justice system, on average, a year earlier than did those therapeutic child care youths who entered the justice system. School reports also indicated that children who did not receive therapeutic treatment had significantly more disciplinary actions in middle to late childhood.

Child Empowerment Services

Daro and McCurdy (1994) reported that evaluations of child-focused educational efforts designed to reduce the likelihood that a child will submit to abuse have had generally positive findings. They emphasized that child-focused educational efforts are not a sufficient approach to reducing maltreatment, but they may help some children. They noted that evaluative data suggests positive outcomes can be enhanced if programs include the following six features.

1. Provide children with behavioral rehearsals of prevention strategies and offer feedback on their performance to facilitate their depiction of their involvement in abusive as well as unpleasant interactions.

2. Develop curricula with a more balanced developmental perspective, tailoring training materials to children's cognitive characteristics and learning abilities.
3. For young children, present the material in stimulating and varied ways to sustain their attention and to reinforce the information learned.
4. Teach generic concepts such as assertive behavior, decision-making skills, and communication skills that children can use in everyday situations, not just to fend off abuse.
5. Repeatedly stress the need for children to tell every time someone continues to touch them in a way that makes them uneasy.
6. Develop longer programs that are better incorporated into regular school curricula and practices. (pp. 415-416)

FACILITATING PARENT-CHILD RELATIONSHIPS

Increasing parents' child management skills may successfully reduce negative parent-child interactions, but such efforts may not significantly improve issues of attachment and positive emotional bonding, or resolve cognitive distortions and negative attitudes regarding parenting and children (Azar, 1997; Wolfe, 1985). Positive, spontaneous interactions and caregiving may still be missing.

Egeland and his colleagues provided a comprehensive review of the research on attachment-based interventions (2000). Their findings indicated that empirical investigations of these approaches are limited in number. Furthermore, the research appears to focus on mothers exclusively, and typically has not specifically targeted maltreated children and their parents.

In their review, Egeland and colleagues (2000) noted that attachment interventions vary in a number of ways, including their goals, methods, participants, and so forth. At their core, however, attachment-based interventions appear to share a common goal of facilitating secure attachment relationships between parent and child.

Egeland and colleagues also noted that while some attachment-based interventions focus directly on the parent-child relationship, other approaches attempt to interrupt the cycle of intergenerational transmission of insecure attachment, poor-quality parenting, and child maltreatment by providing a supportive and corrective therapist-parent relationship designed to help parents resolve the effects of the negative childhood experiences they had with their own parents. These approaches consider the parent-therapist relationship the catalyst for change in the parent-child dyad.

Other attachment-based approaches focus more directly on the parent-child relationship. Although the goals of infant-parent attachment-based interventions generally appear more broadly defined, some interventions are designed specifically to enhance the parents' sensitivity to their child's needs (Egeland et al., 2000). Egeland and colleagues also noted that frequently such approaches provide more emphasis on helping parents better recognize their child's needs, than on strengthening the parent's ability to respond to the child's behaviors and communications.

Hughes (1997) reported that the primary goals of therapy with adopted and foster children who have significant attachment problems is to facilitate the child's attachment to his current parents and promote the development of an integrated sense of self. He asserted that for therapy to be effective the therapist must engage the child at the level of preverbal attunement, not rational discussions. He emphasized that therapy also must involve a lot of physical contact between the child and his or her parent and therapist, especially at times of intense therapeutic work when the child's intense emotions are "received, accepted, and integrated into the self" (p. 7).

Other attachment-based interventions include those that emphasize the importance of providing support for parents through intervention programs while helping parents develop social supports within their environment (Egeland et al., 2000). Egeland and colleagues noted, however, that such interventions commonly have other objectives as well, such as enhancing sensitivity, facilitating parent-child interactions, providing parenting information, and promoting infant development.

As a summary, Egeland and colleagues concluded that

> Based on the research findings regarding breaking the cycle of abuse, as well as theory and research on the development of attachment relationships and inner working models (IWM) of attachment, a number of goals and strategies for preventive interventions emerged. These included: 1) modifying parent's IWM via a trusting relationship with a primary service provider; 2) facilitating healthy resolution of relationship issues from the parent's past; 3) nurturing positive IWN of self

through a strength-focused empowerment approach to both parents and general life management; and 4) facilitating change in sensitivity, perception, and understanding of the baby by providing support, guidance, and information. (p. 62)

This philosophy is reflected in Egeland and his colleagues' prevention and intervention program, Project STEEP (Steps Toward Effective Enjoyable Parenting). This program was designed for mothers who are considered high-risk for parenting difficulties due to poverty. It combined home visits beginning during pregnancy with group interventions. In addition, therapeutic videotaping of interactions between the mother and infant were used. The objectives of this intervention included helping the mother understand how her perceptions, feelings, and interactions with her baby may be related to her own childhood experiences as well as assisting the mother in becoming more sensitive and responsive to her baby's needs and signals. To evaluate the program's effectiveness, 154 pregnant mothers were randomly assigned to a treatment and control group. Follow-up assessments at thirteen and nineteen months indicated mothers in the treatment group had a better understanding of infant development, had better relationships with their infants, exhibited less depression and anxiety, and were more competent in managing their daily lives than the controls. In addition, mothers in the treatment group evidenced improvement in sensitivity, responsivity, and availability to their infants at the thirteen-month follow-up. At nineteen months, however, there were no differences in the percentage of securely attached infants in the treatment and control groups (Egeland et al., 2000).

Egeland and colleagues (2000) hypothesized that the absence of a positive effect of treatment on attachment classifications might be due to several factors. Some mothers may not have been able to benefit from the insight-oriented approach due to behavioral, cognitive, and adjustment problems. He noted that, in retrospect, the mothers with lower intellectual functioning needed more directive teaching of specific and concrete parenting skills and more frequent and intensive interventions than their program could provide.

These authors also pointed out, however, that this problem of enhancing attachment security may be even more difficult because there are many parenting characteristics and behaviors that contribute to the development of a secure attachment. Teaching in one area (e.g., to respond to the child's physical needs) will not necessarily assure that the parent will be *emotionally* responsive to her or his child's needs. They noted that attachment theory suggests unresolved issues from childhood can interfere with the parent's ability to sense and respond to the emotional needs of the infant. They proposed that if this is so, "it would be necessary to change her [or his] expectations regarding emotional openness, vulnerability and trust in relationships in order to promote a secure attachment with her [or his] infant" (p. 69). They pointed out that accomplishing this goal would require insight-oriented therapy. It also would most likely entail lengthy and intensive interventions to develop emotional and behavioral sensitivity and firmly establish more adaptive behavior patterns that are utilized even under stress. Thus, effective interventions may require approaches that facilitate not only the parent's behavioral sensitivity and responsiveness, but also their emotional sensitivity and responsivity.

Based on their literature review, Egeland and his colleagues (2000) concluded research findings suggest that to be effective, intervention programs designed to facilitate parent-child relationships should begin early and be of sufficient duration. They also stressed that interventions need to be tailored to individual family and family members' needs and emphasize natural and community-based supports rather than only therapeutic interventions.

INDIVIDUAL THERAPY AND LONG-TERM THERAPY WITH PARENTS

Conflicting views regarding the usefulness of individual therapy appear in the literature. For example, Cohn and Daro (1987) found that traditional individual psychotherapy was less successful than group or family treatment. In contrast, Grayson (1995) observed that neglectful and economically disadvantaged parents and parents with little education often do not do well when placed in group therapies.

Further research (Egeland et al., 1988) suggests long-term therapy can be instrumental in helping some parents break the intergenerational cycle of maltreatment in high-risk populations. Mothers who broke the cycle were more likely to have participated in extensive therapy and appeared more able to integrate their early experiences as victims of maltreatment into their view of themselves. Egeland and colleagues (2000) concluded that, "mothers who had not worked through difficult childhood memories in a positive, therapeutic manner were acting out the memories by repeating the behaviors in their own parenting" (p. 62). Unfortunately, however, such extensive therapy often may not occur in a time frame that meets the needs of a developing child.

ABUSE-FOCUSED INTERVENTIONS

Physical Abuse

Many studies of parenting interventions have focused on a limited number of treatment targets, such as the parent's child-rearing knowledge, skills, and behavior; impulse and anger management; stress management; and parental problem-solving skills (Schellenbach, 1998). In the area of physical abuse, interventions focused on helping parents reduce physiological reactivity, improve anger management, and develop enhanced empathy with their children. Schellenbach reviewed studies and found parents reported improved relationships with their children, less anger and reactivity, and fewer symptoms of depression following interventions. Improvements in the parents' attitudes toward their children were not maintained at follow-up; however, there were no significant changes in certain targeted behaviors, such as coercive commands by parents and playful interactions.

Behavioral interventions have included a variety of techniques such as coaching and modeling of appropriate parenting behaviors, role-playing, homework assignments, and feedback. Studies have reported improved parent-child interactions, greater child compliance, and less parental reliance on corporal punishment (Wolfe, 1994). Similarly, cognitive interventions that emphasized cognitive restructuring, problem-solving training, techniques to enhance coping (such as relaxation training and self-management skills), and anger management also have reported positive results, with programs that have combined cognitive and behavioral interventions, suggesting that an integrated approach may be most effective (Wolfe, 1994).

In one of the few comparative studies to date, Kolko (1996) compared the effectiveness of cognitive-behavioral treatment (CBT), family therapy (FT), and routine community services (RCS) for fifty-five physically abused children and their parents or guardians. Forty-three of the families were randomly assigned to the CBT or FT comparison groups. Twelve other families, who could not be randomized, were referred to treatment providers in the community.

The CBT groups received parallel parent and child interventions totaling approximately eighteen hours of service each. The children's treatment focused on such issues as family violence and stressors, coping (e.g., safety and support planning and relaxation training), and training in interpersonal skills associated with social competence. The parents' treatment focused on similar issues, including their attitudes concerning family violence and physical punishment, their attributions toward and expectations of their children, and their self-control and child behavior management skills. The FT group promoted family cooperation and motivation through developing an understanding of coercive behavior, enhancing positive communication, and problem-solving skills. The RCS group received treatment, as mandated by their caseworkers, from community providers not involved in the study. These services involved home visits to provide information and support, family skills specialist interventions that provided homemaking and other related interventions, and parenting information and support groups. Some of these interventions were intensive, involving up to twenty hours per week for as long as three months, while others were limited to once or twice a week indefinitely.

Weekly reports of indicators associated with maltreatment were obtained from children and their parents or guardians. These indicators included reports of parental anger, physical discipline or force, and family problems. Measures also included official records of child abuse and other assessment tools such as the Conflict Tactics Scale (CTS) (Straus as cited in Kolko, 1996) and the Child Abuse Potential Inventory (Milner as cited in Kolko, 1996).

Families involved in CBT and FT, in contrast to the RCS comparison group, showed greater improvements in child abuse potential and individual problems, children's externalizing behaviors, parental general distress, family cohesion, and parent-reported child-to-parent violence. FT was associated with greater improvements on child-reported parent-to-child violence as well. CBT and FT interventions also tended to demonstrate more improvement than RCS on certain changes that were observed over time, such as improvements in parent-to-child violence, child internalizing and externalizing problems, and parental depression. Although official records indicated a relatively higher rate of recidivism among RCS subjects (30 percent [three cases]) than CBT (5 percent [one case]) or FT (6 percent [one case]), the cases were few and thus the finding was not statistically significant. Although CBT and FT appeared superior on a number of measures, greater improvements among participants in the RCS group were found in some areas, such as in less general family dysfunction.

In a subsequent report of this study, Kolko (1998) also observed that between 20 percent of the children and 23 percent of the parents independently reported that high levels of physical discipline or force occurred during the early and late phases of treatment, although reportedly few incidents appeared to result in injuries. Reports indicated that an even larger number of subjects experienced increased parental anger and family problems at these times. Parent and child reports that occurred early in treatment predicted reports that occurred late in treatment; however, only the parents' reports were associated with validity measures. Kolko noted that these findings suggest the importance of monitoring such emotions and behaviors routinely throughout treatment.

In his 1996 summary of this research, Kolko (1996) pointed out that the findings of this study are consistent with other findings in the sexual abuse field that support the use of abuse-specific interventions. He also observed that the CBT and FT interventions both utilized "direct and comparable" child and parent interventions (p. 339) and suggested that integrating individual and family influences during treatment, as well as supports outside the family, may further enhance interventions.

As in other areas, the provision of multiple, diverse services to children and their parents who have been abusive make it difficult to determine what makes the difference. Kolko (1998) commented that because there have been so few studies pertaining to the treatment of child victims of physical abuse, conclusions about the efficacy of these interventions are tentative. Most programs have limited their focus to preschoolers and measures of improvements in developmental skills, self-concept, and peer relationships. In addition, the work to date is illuminating but studies with improved methodologies, follow-ups, and comparative analyses of different treatment interventions are still needed.

Neglect

Because poverty is very strongly associated with neglect (Sedlack and Broadhurst, 1996), interventions may require efforts to provide for families' basic needs.

> Services may include the following: (a) emergency financial assistance, (b) low-cost housing, (c) emergency food and clothing, (d) free or low-cost medical care, (e) transportation, (f) homemaker/home management aides, (g) low-cost child care, (h) mental health assessment and treatment, (i) temporary foster care, (j) budget/credit counseling, (k) job training and placement, (l) parent support/skills training, and (m) recreation programs for children and parents. (Gaudin, 1993, pp. 70-71)

It is hoped that by mobilizing these practical services and resources, the parent's resistance, feelings of hopelessness, and distrust of professionals may be reduced.

However, as Catwell (1997) noted, most people who live in poverty are very adequate parents. Furthermore, interventions designed to remediate socioeconomic factors associated with child neglect have not succeeded in improving families' socioeconomic status or reducing neglectful behaviors (Crittenden, 1999). Crittenden pointed out, "it may be that although economic factors often contribute to neglect, they are neither necessary nor sufficient to cause neglect" (p. 48). Thus, although economic problems may coexist with neglect, other factors contribute to it.

Parents who are neglectful have been described as frequently showing a lack of psychological maturity, often related to a lack of nurturing when they were children (Gaudin, 1993). They also have been found to be self-focused, impulsive, and lack the wherewithal to organize their lives to meet their own needs, let alone the needs of their children. For parents to learn to nurture their children, they are likely to require nurturing themselves. "Intervention with neglectful parents requires that the professional helper 'parent the parent' before they are able to nurture successfully" (Gaudin, 1993, p. 71). In addition, treatment goals will need to include helping the parents develop feelings of hope, self-esteem, and self-efficacy.

Research specifically focusing on treatment outcomes with parents who have neglected their children, and with children who have been neglected, is very limited. As with all studies in the area of child maltreatment, the few existing studies have methodological problems. Findings from these studies have not been encouraging. Daro (1988) reviewed nineteen child maltreatment demonstration intervention projects, four of which were designed to intervene specifically in cases involving child neglect. Another eleven addressed the full range of child maltreatment. Daro found that, of the neglect cases, 66 percent were known to have new occurrences of maltreatment during the intervention period. As in other types of maltreatment, the severity of the initial maltreatment was associated with poorer outcomes. In cases of neglect, substance abuse appeared especially problematic for facilitating treatment progress. In spite of these discouraging findings, some approaches were more effective than other approaches.

While noting that strong empirical support for specific interventions is lacking, DePanfilis (1999) observed that experience suggests guiding principles for intervention. She stressed the importance of beginning interventions with a comprehensive family assessment. Following this assessment,

> promising interventions are directed to developing or providing concrete resources, social support, developmental remediation, cognitive or behavioral interventions, individual oriented interventions, and family-focused interventions. Services are geared to empower families to access the resources needed to manage the multiple stresses and strains in their lives so that they may provide children with adequate care and guidance. It is also essential that the services are available to help children overcome developmental deficits that may have resulted from chronic inattention to their needs. (p. 229)

Behavioral interventions appear to be successful in teaching some neglecting parents home management skills, parent-child interactions, and meal preparation (Gaudin, 1993; Grayson, 1995). Important treatment components include relevant, clearly defined, achievable, and agreed-upon short-range goals. In addition, it appears necessary to use a broad range of services from multiple sources that use a variety of intervention methods, such as a combination of parenting groups and individual in-home services, in order to improve informal social networks and daily living skill deficits. As noted with parents with mental retardation (McConnell et al., 1997), interventions should be designed to accommodate clients' learning styles and difficulties.

Gaudin (1993) noted that short-term interventions have not, however, been successful. Grayson (1995) noted long-term treatment of at least twelve to eighteen months might be required. Crittenden (1996) reported that neglectful parents might require extended services, lasting two to five years or more. She observed that many neglectful parents have limited abilities to respond to interventions that require fast change or appreciable intellectual capabilities. They also are likely to become overwhelmed if too many interventions are offered concurrently.

Programs that address neglect typically emphasize parent interventions, whereas infant stimulation programs and therapeutic day care are designed to compensate for the lack of care these children receive from their parents. Infant stimulation programs have been found to be effective for neglected and physically abused children (Crittenden, 1996; Gaudin, 1993). A few other programs provided children and teenagers with skill-based interventions, temporary housing, and support groups as part of a comprehensive approach to treatment (Gaudin, 1993; Kolko, 1998). School- and community-based programs also may help remedy the negative effects of neglect in children. Examples of such programs include Big Brothers Big Sisters of America, whose volunteers provide mentoring, nurturing, tutoring, and social support to youths. Research has shown these programs are effective at reducing violent crime, aggression, and substance abuse among youths (Mihaic et al., 2001).

In reviewing literature pertaining to child maltreatment interventions, Gaudin (1993) observed that the limited information available suggests that direct interventions to ameliorate the negative effects of neglect on children appear to be more effective than parent-focused interventions.

Crittenden (1999) proposed that information-processing problems contribute to child neglect by interfering with the parents' ability to accurately understand reality and develop effective problem-solving strategies. She hypothesized that effective interventions would require strategies that address the parent's information processing difficulties.

To illustrate her theory, Crittenden (1999) identified three types of neglect that she called (1) disorganized neglect, (2) emotional neglect, and (3) depressed neglect. She argued that in the disorganized type of neglect the parents' style of information processing emphasizes affect and cognition is minimized. These families may appear crisis prone. In addition, the parents do not take care of their children in a timely or predictable fashion.

In contrast, in the emotionally neglecting group affect is minimized and cognitive approaches to organizing information are stressed. In these families the physical and material needs of the children tend to be met, but their emotional needs are not. Crittenden (1999) noted that financial factors might not be an issue in these families; in fact they may be economically advantaged.

In the third classification, depressed neglect, both cognitive and affective approaches for processing information are shut down. The parent does not interact with the world in general and does not attend to or respond to his or her children's needs.

Crittenden (1999) emphasized that although this model is theoretical, this conceptualization suggests the importance of assessing parental information-processing strategies in cases of child neglect. She maintained that, in order for interventions to be effective, approaches will need to be responsive to how these parents process the information that is provided to assure that it is not blocked out and its meaning is understood. Furthermore, Crittenden noted that for interventions to be effective, "they must change how information is processed and used to organize behavior by individuals. This will require systematic and deliberate consideration of *how* specific interventions function and *who* is likely to benefit (a) at what time, (b) with which combination and order of techniques, and (c) in what context" (pp. 65-66).

Sexual Abuse

Treatment of Children Who Have Been Sexually Abused

Abuse-specific interventions with children who have been sexually abused usually involve a psychoeducational component in combination with cognitive-behavioral interventions. Components typically include

> educating children and parents about the nature of child sexual abuse and offenders, encouraging the expression of a range of abuse-related feelings, identifying and correcting distorted

cognitions, teaching anxiety management, gradual exposure to memories of the abuse experience, promoting abuse-response skills, and providing support. (Berliner, 1997, p. 170)

Support for these interventions is provided by studies in this area (e.g., Reeker et al., 1997). However, research on treatment approaches with children who have been abused is in its infancy and, as is generally true of like research throughout the child maltreatment field, methodological problems exist (Finkelhor and Berliner, 1995). In spite of these difficulties, however, the results of various studies suggest cognitive-behavioral interventions that focus on the abuse and related emotions appear particularly promising (Berliner and Saunders, 1996; Cohen and Mannarino, 1997; Deblinger et al., 1996).

As an example of such research, Cohen and Mannarino (1997) randomly assigned sexually abused preschoolers to cognitive-behavioral treatment (CBT) or nondirective supportive therapy (NST). CBT was significantly more effective than NST in reducing behavior problems, internalizing symptoms, and sexually inappropriate behaviors. Improvements were maintained during the year follow-up.

Subsequently, Cohen and Mannarino (1998) randomly assigned sexually abused children ages seven to fourteen to cognitive-behavioral treatment (CBT) or nondirective supportive therapy (NST). Again the children in the CBT group demonstrated improvements in depressive symptomology. In addition, a much greater number of children from the NST group required removal from the program due to persistent inappropriate sexual behavior. The relatively high dropout rate of subjects in the NST group limited the study's power to detect statistical significance between groups.

Group therapy approaches often are used with children who have been sexually abused. The effectiveness of group interventions in comparison to other approaches, however, has not been established (Berliner, 1997). The involvement of a nonabusive parent in the treatment process has been found to facilitate positive outcomes and, for school-aged children, parental involvement alone has not been found to be as effective as interventions that involve both the parent and the child (Cohen and Mannarino, 1997; Deblinger et al., 1996). Parental involvement may provide parents with the needed information and skills to help their child effectively resolve the sexually abusive experience (Berliner, 1997).

Outcome studies of sex-abuse-specific treatment with children suggest that positive results can be achieved in a relatively short time when structured, time-limited, cognitive behavioral interventions are employed (Berliner and Saunders, 1996; Cohen and Mannarino, 1997; Deblinger et al., 1996). However, children who have been sexually abused differ in a variety of ways and sex abuse does not need to "become the defining event of a lifetime or leave children with residual problems" (Berliner, 1997, p. 171). Because of this variability among children and the possible range of symptom expression (from an absence of symptoms to multiple problems) it is "unlikely that any one particular therapy is going to be suitable or effective for all children" (Finkelhor and Berliner, 1995, p. 1416). Furthermore, it is important to remember that many of these children and their families frequently experience a myriad of difficulties.

> [O]verfocusing on the sexual abuse or failing to recognize the contribution of other factors to the difficulties of sexually abused children may exaggerate the significance of the sexual abuse in the larger context of troubled children's lives and miss other important targets for therapeutic interventions. (Berliner, 1997, p. 163)

To effectively intervene in the lives of multiply abused, stressed, and disadvantaged children and their families, other approaches and longer-term therapies may be required.

Treatment with Individuals Who Have Sexually Offended

As in other areas of child maltreatment, early approaches to treating people who have been sexually abusive involved psychodynamic and psychoanalytic approaches. Studies evaluating the effectiveness of these approaches have been limited by methodological problems and available research efforts do not generally support these methods (Becker and Murphy, 1998; Marshall and Barbaree, 1990).

Feminist theories have emphasized negative aspects of male socialization in the development of sexual violence against women. These views have received some support (Becker and Murphy, 1998). Becker and Murphy reported that some studies have identified an association between sexual aggression and sexual stereotyping, the acceptance of rape myths, and hostile attitudes toward women (Malamuth et al., 1991). Biological theories also have received some attention, as demonstrated by explorations of the role of neurotransmitters in modulating sexual behavior (Kafka, 1997).

Cognitive-behavioral theories are in the forefront. These theories consider sexual aggression to result from the conditioning of deviant sexual arousal and the development of cognitive distortions that justify and maintain the abusive behavior (Becker and Murphy, 1998). Currently, most practitioners who work in this area employ cognitive-behavioral interventions involving a relapse prevention model with selected pharmacological approaches used when appropriate (Becker and Murphy, 1998; Murphy and Smith, 1996).

In their review of treatment programs, Marshall and Barbaree (1990) noted that programs differ in terms of the intensity of therapeutic contact, the duration of treatment, and expected progress. They indicated that, in spite of these differences, there is agreement that the primary treatment components are (1) sexual behaviors and interests, (2) a variety of social difficulties, and (3) cognitive distortions about the offending behavior.

Reviews of treatment approaches with adults (Becker and Murphy, 1998; Grossman et al., 1999; Murphy and Smith, 1996) as well as juveniles (Becker and Hunter, 1997; Bourke and Donohue, 1996; National Adolescent Perpetrator Network [NAPN], 1993), indicate that sex-offense-specific programs typically use interventions that target risk factors associated with sexual abuse. These frequently include interventions that are designed to do the following:

- Resolve cognitive distortions regarding sexual abuse and rape
- Resolve other relevant cognitive distortions such as negative attitudes toward girls and women
- Promote positive attitudes and provide accurate information about human sexuality
- Develop techniques for reducing and managing deviant arousal fantasies and patterns
- Strengthen appropriate arousal
- Increase social competence (e.g., social and dating skills, anger management, and personal hygiene) and reduce procriminal attitudes
- Resolve personal victimization issues
- Develop victim empathy

- Address family difficulties and dysfunction
- Enhance self-efficacy and self-esteem
- Establish lifestyle changes to reduce access to potential victims
- Promote relapse prevention

Research findings (Rotheram-Borus et al., 1991) that adolescents who have sexually offended are especially deficient in their general knowledge about AIDS and safe sex practices as compared to a runaway comparison group, suggest that this is another area that requires intervention.

One other common goal of treatment is the reduction of denial and minimization (Chaffin and Bonner, 1998). However, research findings generally have not demonstrated that denying offenses is associated with sexual reoffending in adults (Hanson and Bussière, 1998) or juveniles (Hunter and Figueredo, 1999).

Research with juveniles (Miner and Crimmins, 1995) and adults (Marshall et al., 2000) has also identified social isolation from positive interactions with peers and families as an area that warrants intervention. Consequently, interventions that promote positive family relationships, positive school attachments in youths, and facilitate positive emotional attachments in general are considered appropriated treatment goals.

Other relevant interventions in this area are similar to those employed in other comprehensive interventions in the broader range of child maltreatment cases. These include strategies to enhance impulse control and facilitate good judgment; improve academic, vocational, and basic living skills; resolve personal victimization experiences; address coexisting disorders or difficulties; resolve family dysfunction and impaired sibling relationships; develop prosocial relationships with peers; and encourage positive sexual development and identity (Becker and Hunter, 1997; Becker and Murphy, 1998; Bourke and Donohue, 1996; Marshall et al., 2000; Murphy and Smith, 1996; NAPN, 1993). When people who have been sexually abusive are parents, interventions designed to promote safe and positive parenting in general also are required.

Psychopharmocological interventions, such as sex-drive reducing medications such as medroxyprogesterone, have also been used in treating sexual offenders. These medications have been found to be effective in reducing sex offending in some adult offenders (Greenberg and Bradford, 1997; Grossman et al., 1999; Prentky, 1997) and may be used as part of a comprehensive treatment intervention. Some of these medications (e.g., antiandrogen drugs) can have serious side effects, however, including negative effect on normal development and growth. In view of such side effects, there are substantial ethical concerns related to the use of such medications with youths (Hunter and Lexier, 1998).

More recently the class of antidepressants called selective serotonin reuptake inhibitors (SSRIs) has been found to be useful with some adults and juveniles who sexually offend, again when used as part of a comprehensive treatment intervention (Hunter and Lexier, 1998; Greenberg and Bradford, 1997; Prentky, 1997). Yet, many basic questions concerning psychopharmocological approaches remain, including who is likely to benefit from such an approach and at what dosages (Hunter and Lexier, 1998).

For theoretical reasons, group therapies are frequently thought to be the treatment of choice when working with people who have sexually offended, and cotherapist teams, preferably involving a female and male therapist, often are recommended (Marshall and Barbaree, 1990; Murphy and Smith, 1996; NAPN, 1993). Group therapy is likely to be cost-effective when presenting educational information to multiple offenders and may facilitate new ways of thinking and social interaction that are unavailable in traditional individualized treatment. In addition, male-female teams can model egalitarian relationships between the sexes. Yet, regarding male-female cotherapist teams, as Murphy and Smith (1996) noted, "there is no empirical evidence to suggest that this is necessary, and in many small programs this luxury cannot be afforded" (p. 185). In addition, there is no empirical evidence to suggest that group therapies are superior to other approaches (Chaffin and Bonner, 1998; Murphy and Smith, 1996; NAPN, 1993; Weinrott, 1996). Furthermore, negative peer associations that result from treatment (before, during, or after group sessions) may be harmful, especially for young adolescents (Dishion et al., 1999).

Maletzky (1999) also noted that claims that group therapy is more effective for reducing sex offending are not empirically supported. He acknowledged that group sex offender treatment may be especially beneficial for "*some* offenders and for *some* of their goals" (p. 181) and, as examples, noted that this may be so for reducing denial and possibly for providing a positive modeling effect. However, his point remained that the effectiveness of these objectives in reducing sex offending has not been demonstrated.

In addition, Maletzky (1999) reported that there are several studies demonstrating that cognitive-behavioral therapy provided in an individual therapy format was more effective than when it was provided in group therapy; although as with most studies, this research was retrospective, uncontrolled, and limited geographically. He argued that, "Providing one-to-one therapy is time-consuming, labor-intensive, and expensive, yet it offers an unparalleled opportunity to explore individual parameters of relapse prevention and to decondition idiosyncratic patterns of arousal not possible in a group setting. It offers the advantages of more personal and intensive treatment and the opportunity to reassess continually how each patient is progressing" (p. 180).

In addition to more traditional therapeutic approaches, Murphy and Smith (1996) emphasized that treatment efforts must also extend outside the therapist's office. They argued, "Optimal treatment requires close monitoring in the community by probation or parole personnel and/or significant others who are aware of risk factors and who are willing to coordinate their monitoring with the treatment provider" (p. 185).

Balancing the areas of consensus in the field of sexual offending treatment is other research (Barbaree et al., 1994; Knight and Prentky, 1990) that reminds practitioners that people who engage in sexually aggressive behavior are a heterogeneous group with varying reasons for their abusive behavior. Therefore, treatment programs also need to consider a wider range of individual factors and be responsive to individual differences (Becker and Murphy, 1998).

Furthermore, regarding juveniles who have sexually offended, there is a question as to whether these youths need to be treated differently from youths who engage in other forms of criminal behaviors (Lab et al., 1993). Jacobs and colleagues (1997), noting the absence of significant differences in the research literature between groups of juvenile sex offenders and juveniles who committed other types of offenses concluded, "The similarities are indicative of commensurate therapeutic needs for both types of offenders" (p. 201).

As Milloy (1994) pointed out, juvenile sex offender treatment typically includes interventions that may be appropriate for juvenile offenders in general, such as social skills, sex education, anger management, accepting responsibility for one's offenses, and victim empathy.

She argued, "the segregation of juvenile sex offenders is a costly approach whose worth is unproven" (p. 10).

Whether youths who have been sexually abusive should be mainstreamed with youths who have committed other types of offenses or youths who have behavior problems but have not been charged with juvenile offenses remains a complex question. Clearly, other factors, such as the safety of all of the youths, including those who have sexually offended and may be targeted because of their sex offending histories, must be considered when designing appropriate treatments and treatment settings. The heterogeneity of youths who have sexually offended "suggests that no single treatment regime will be effective in all cases" (Kavoussi et al., 1988, p. 243). A one-size fits-all approach can be costly and may be harmful to the youth and his or her family (Becker, 1998). As Chaffin and Bonner (1998) have pointed out, "perhaps it is time to emphasize some flexibility and compassion in which treatments we choose and to which individual youngsters we apply them and to realize that individual need, not dogma, should dictate what must be accomplished" (p. 316).

The importance of tailoring interventions to individual needs was exemplified by Pithers and colleagues' (1998) work with children who had sexual behavior problems. These researchers identified five subtypes of children with sexual behavior problems: (1) sexually aggressive, (2) nonsymptomatic, (3) highly traumatized, (4) abusive reactive, and (5) rule breaker. They found there were some differences between how children in various subtype classifications responded to different types of treatment.

At intake the children and their families were randomly assigned to one of two thirty-two-week treatment conditions. One modality involved expressive therapy. The other was a modified form of relapse prevention. Both approaches involved nonabusive parents in parallel group interventions. The Child Sexual Behavior Inventory-3 (CSBI-3) (Friedrich, 1997) was utilized to measure progress. Results indicated that most child types evidenced similar degrees of change regardless of treatment modality.

The results of this research found that a slightly larger number of the sexually aggressive children in the expressive therapy, compared with those in the modified relapse prevention therapy, evidenced reduced levels of sexual behavior problems. These findings were tempered, however, by the fact that a similar number of the sexually aggressive children in the expressive therapy actually had increased rates of sexual behavior problems. The highly traumatized children, on the other hand, did significantly better after the first sixteen weeks of treatment with the modified relapse prevention treatment than the expressive therapy. In fact, highly traumatized children who were in the expressive therapy evidenced a slight increase in sexualized behavior.

The results of this research also showed that, while some child types responded well to some type of treatment, others did not. For example, more than half of the highly traumatized children evidenced significant reductions in problematic sexual behavior after the first sixteen weeks of treatment. In contrast, only 7 percent of the sexually aggressive children had significant decreases in their sexual behavior problems regardless of treatment approach, suggesting the children classified as sexually aggressive may need more intensive treatment than they received through the research study.

Lastly, there has been continuing debate as to whether treatment interventions with sexual offenders are really effective at all in reducing sexual offending (Marshall and Pithers, 1994; Quinsey et al., 1993). Reviews of the treatment outcome research suggest studies that have shown negative treatment outcomes have been marred by methodological problems and antiquated treatment approaches (Marshall and Pithers, 1994). Although more recent studies are not free from methodological difficulties, participants in more modern programs have demonstrated lower reoffense rates than untreated offenders and other comparison groups (Becker and Murphy, 1998; Grossman et al., 1999; Hall, 1995; Marshall and Pithers, 1994; Worling and Curren, 2000). As is consistent with the heterogeneity of this population, some programs may be more effective with certain groups of offenders and less effective with others, such as exhibitionists and rapists (Marshall and Barbaree, 1990).

Partner Abuse

Adult Interventions

As noted in Chapter 3, partner violence has been found to co-occur with child maltreatment. Studies have found that between one-third and three-quarters of men who assault their wives also physically abuse their children (Bowker et al., 1988; Jaffe et al., 1990; Saunders,

1995). In addition, some batterers also rape their partners (Campbell and Alford, 1989). Severe and frequent partner abuse has been associated with more severe child abuse (Bowker et al., 1988). When partner violence is present, specialized interventions to address this form of violence may be a necessary part of an individualized, comprehensive intervention.

Adults Who Have Assaulted Their Partners

Individuals who abuse their partners are a heterogeneous group (Grayson, 1996). As appears true in other areas of family and general violence, research findings suggest there may be a small group, including individuals with substance abuse disorders, severe psychopathology, and antisocial personality disorders, who are responsible for most of the recidivism in this area. As in these other areas, individualized interventions may be needed to maximize the effectiveness of partner abuse interventions.

Interventions for men who abuse their partners have multiplied significantly during the last two decades. Interventions for women who are abusive appear to be relatively few. Interventions and programs vary to different degrees in terms of their philosophies, comprehensiveness, duration, and approach (Gondolf, 1999). Most partner abuse intervention programs utilize group interventions and cognitive-behavioral approaches (White and Gondolf, 2000). Interventions may include anger management training, skill building that addresses interpersonal deficits or excesses, resocialization to correct for beliefs that support attitudes of male dominance, and personal accountability for abusive behavior (Gondolf, 1999; White and Gondolf, 2000). Programs may emphasize different interventions depending on their philosophical orientation, structure, and approach (Gondolf, 1993).

Edleson and Syers (1991) randomly assigned 283 men to one of six group treatment formats involving either an education, self-help, or a combined approach and an intensity of either twelve or thirty-two sessions. At an eighteen-month follow-up, there were no significant differences in reassault rates between the twelve or thirty-two session groups. Nearly two-thirds of the men who completed the education and combined groups, and who were found at follow-up, were described as nonviolent since treatment. Rates of nonviolence were even higher for participants who completed the self-help group and were available at the eighteen-month follow-up. This finding contrasted with the six-month follow-up, when this group had the highest recidivism rate; however, it is possible that some of those who were not available at follow-up had been violent. Court involvement and no previous mental health treatment were associated with a lower likelihood of violence at the eighteen-month follow-up.

Similarly, Gondolf (1999) reported results from a comparative study of four geographic areas' approaches to partner abuse. The findings suggest the interventions used appeared to contribute to a short-term cessation of partner violence in most participants. The interventions varied in terms of whether services were pre- or posttrial, the program's duration (three to nine months), and whether additional services were provided (in-house alcohol treatment and occasional referrals). Outcome measures revealed no significant differences across setting in the reassault rate, the number of men who made threats, and the victim's reported quality of life. However, the longest and most comprehensive program showed significantly lower rates of severe reassaults. Gondolf hypothesized that the in-house alcohol treatment program might explain this result because alcohol abuse is associated with severe violence.

Gondolf also reported that each of the intervention systems in his study were well-established batterers' programs that complied to state standards that require batterer accountability for their abuse, exposing and not accepting rationalizations for their abusive behaviors, and identifying the assault of women as a means of power and control.

Programs also collaborated with women's service programs and the criminal justice system. He noted that these factors might be fundamental contributions to program effectiveness. He also noted, however, that the effectiveness of one program in a specific community does not mean that a similar program would be effective in a different community.

Saunders (1996) used random assignment to compare a cognitive-behavioral didactic batterers' therapy group with a psychodynamic therapy group. The reassault rates and other outcome measures such as the women's level of fear and perceived changes in the men were approximately the same for each group. However, men with certain characteristics tended to fare better if assigned to a particular treatment modality: men with dependent personalities did better if they were in the psychodynamic group, whereas men who had more anti-social characteristics had better outcomes if they were in the cogni-tive-behavioral group.

The wide differences in how partner violence is understood are perhaps best exemplified in the controversy about when and whether couples' counseling is appropriate when partner violence has oc-curred (Berliner, 1996; Gondolf, 1993). Concerns about conjoint in-terventions primarily focus on the victim's safety. Questions include whether the perpetrator may retaliate for disclosures made in treat-ment, whether the context of the conjoint sessions will contribute to the victim feeling or being blamed for her perceived role in marital difficulties, and whether reconciliation with the perpetrator is even in the woman's best interest (Gondolf, 1993). Some practitioners have argued strongly against the use of couples' counseling in any such cases.

In contrast, O'Leary (1996) has argued that there are no singular answers to complex problems such as partner violence. O'Leary has pointed out that individuals who engage in such behaviors are a di-verse group and that the severity of violence ranges as well. Citing re-search that 89 percent of individuals in physically aggressive rela-tionships have reported that a lack of communication is the most significant problem they experience, he argues that couples' therapy should be considered as one approach for such individuals. He has also noted that marital discord is a strong risk factor for partner abuse and questions whether providers may be ethically remiss in not pro-viding treatment for the couple, at some point, when a woman wants to remain with her partner.

O'Leary also emphasized, however, that his approach to partner abuse is not traditional couples' therapy but rather

> a structured treatment that focuses on the following: (a) eliminat-ing psychological and physical violence, (b) accepting responsi-bility for the escalation of angry interchanges, (c) recognizing and controlling self-angering thoughts, (d) communicating more effectively, (e) increasing caring and mutually pleasurable ac-tivities, and (f) understanding that each partner has the right to be treated with respect. (pp. 451-452)

He noted that men who have engaged in extreme forms of violence and whose wives are fearful about remaining in the relationship or this form of intervention are excluded from couples' therapy at his clinic. He reported that research has supported the effectiveness of his approach for reducing physical and psychological aggression and enhancing marital satisfaction.

Others also have suggested that couples' therapy may be a valid technique in some cases of partner abuse (Gondolf, 1993; Grayson, 1996). Grayson has pointed out that couples' therapies are based on systems and learning theory.

> Systems theory states that all parts of the system must respond when one part changes, thus involving both partners may be necessary for change. Similarly, learning theory considers cues, rewards, and responses important to maintaining behaviors. If both parties learn different responses, new learning patterns can be better reinforced. (pp. 12, 14)

Gondolf (1993) suggested that when couples' therapy is employed, it might be best to introduce it after the completion of a batterers' intervention program and at least six to twelve months of no violence. He has also noted, however, that couples' interventions may be ineffective and even dangerous with people who are antisocial psychopathic.

Clinicians appear to agree that couples' therapy is not appropriate when it would jeopardize the safety of the victim, when the violence has been severe or frequent, when the perpetrator is chemically dependent or has mental illness, or when the victim does not want couples' therapy (Grayson, 1996). Grayson also states that if couples' sessions are implemented, safeguards such as individual sessions to monitor victim safety should be in place.

Adults Who Have Been Abused

The individual treatment needs of those who have been assaulted may be very relevant for the prevention of child maltreatment. A detailed discussion of that literature is beyond the scope of this guide.

In recent years, because of the co-occurrence of child maltreatment and partner assault, there have been increasing efforts to provide interventions to children and their mothers who have experienced partner assault (Edleson, 1999a). Recently, a special issue of the journal *Child Maltreatment* focused specifically on this topic (Edleson, 1999b). In his introduction to the section Model Programs and Interventions, Edleson reported that in 1998, the National Council of Juvenile and Family Court Judges published a review of over thirty programs titled *Family Violence: Emerging Programs for Battered Mothers and Their Children.* Three additional programs are described in this special issue of *Child Maltreatment.* The goals of such programs typically include helping mothers and children live safely after leaving shelters and improving the collaboration among child protection agencies, the courts, and battered women's advocates when children have been abused and neglected.

Collaborative approaches appear much needed in this area. Frequently child protective workers and battered women's advocates have been at odds (Findlater and Kelley, 1999). Advocates have perceived child protective workers as insensitive to the difficulties experienced by battered mothers. Meanwhile, child protective workers have perceived advocates as unconcerned with the safety of the children when mothers appear unable to adequately protect their children from violence.

Such black-and-white thinking is simplistic and ignores the varying and complex needs of the individuals involved. Some parents who have been abused by their partners maltreat their children (Saunders, 1995). It is likely that abused parents also differ in their ability to adequately protect their children, and the types of interventions that may be required to improve their protective capacity vary as well. Individualized assessments and interventions may better address these complex issues and help provide for the safety of children and their abused parent as well as the developmental needs of exposed and often abused and neglected children.

Child Interventions

As noted in Chapter 2, research studies have demonstrated that exposing children to family violence can have serious consequences for their psychosocial development, even when children are not directly abused. For some children, being exposed to partner abuse may be as harmful to the child's healthy development as being the one abused (Jaffe et al., 1990). When children have been exposed to partner and family violence specialized interventions to help them process their experience and reactions are required (Jaffe and Geffner, 1998). Individualized assessments and interventions are needed.

Structured treatment groups that use psychoeducational and cognitive-behavioral approaches have been developed as interventions for children who have been exposed to family violence (Kolko, 1998; Sudermann and Jaffe, 1997). Age appropriate interventions are applied and emphasize identifying feelings, safety skills, prosocial conflict management skills, social support, self-concept and social competence, not assuming responsibility for parent violence, and so forth. The few existing evaluations of this approach suggest that these groups may help children develop safety skills, assign appropriate responsibility for the violence, strengthen self-esteem, develop improved perceptions of their parents, and become better at separating their feelings of love for their parents and their rejection of parental violent behaviors. These findings are limited by common methodological problems (Kolko, 1998; Sudermann and Jaffe, 1997). Other issues, such as post-traumatic stress symptoms that occur as a result of the exposure to violence, may need to be addressed in individual therapy (Kolko, 1998).

PARENTS WITH MENTAL RETARDATION

Tymchuk and colleagues (1990) found that parents with mental retardation can be trained to recognize home dangers and implement precautions. The results of interventions, however, were variable and obtaining positive results required much time. In addition, periodic training sessions may be required for the parents to maintain learned skills. Tymchuk and Feldman (1991) found maintenance of skills has not been consistent and difficulties considering positive alternatives may occur in the heat of the moment.

Training programs for parents with mental retardation must be specially designed and implemented by individuals trained to work with this population. Performance-based parent training strategies, such as task analysis, modeling, role playing, feedback, and reinforced practice with tangible reinforcement tend to be most effective, and may be more effective than verbal therapies. Successful training outcomes for parents with mental retardation may be thwarted by problems, such as depression, chronic medical difficulties, and insufficient supports.

Children of mentally retarded parents may benefit from specialized early interventions (Tymchuk and Feldman, 1991). Interventions may include therapeutic day treatment programs as well as psychological and special educational services outside the home.

SUBSTANCE ABUSE

As in other areas, substance abuse issues require individualized approaches that are likely to be helpful to the individual client in decreasing the risk of substance abusing behaviors. Miller and colleagues (1995) conducted an extensive metanalysis of the alcohol abuse outcome literature. The modalities described as effective and having the strongest effects included brief interventions that typically focus on less severe abuse problems and that frequently involve screening assessments and motivational enhancement strategies. Strong positive effects also were found for motivational enhancement, community reinforcement, behavioral contracting, disulfiram, behavioral self-control training, and social skills training that focused on life problem areas considered related to drinking and relapse, but not specifically on alcohol consumption. Some mild positive effects were found for a self-help manual, behavioral marital and family therapy, lithium, and electrical aversion therapy. In contrast, approaches not found to be very effective included general alcohol counseling, educational lectures and films, general psychotherapy, confrontational counseling, relaxation training, and antianxiety medication. Two studies found Alcoholics Anonymous was not effective when clients were required to attend by external forces.

MENTAL HEALTH INTERVENTIONS

Mental health problems and psychiatric difficulties may need to be addressed before, during, after, or throughout other abuse-focused interventions. For example, Crittenden (1999) indicated that depression is a significant factor for some parents and requires appropriate treatment.

RELAPSE PREVENTION

Relapse prevention (RP) is an approach to treatment that is designed to help clients maintain treatment gains and prevent relapse following treatment (Becker and Murphy, 1998; Hall et al., 1993; Pithers et al., 1987, 1993). RP emphasizes self-management. It requires individuals to identify factors that increase their risk of offending and use strategies to avoid high-risk situations or manage them when they occur. These strategies include self-management approaches as well as the utilization of external strategies, such as the provision of support and supervision by probation or parole officers, family members, or other appropriate members of the community (Becker and Murphy, 1998).

RP initially was designed to help substance abusers prevent reoccurences of substance abusing behavior, and then was applied to sex offenders to reduce sexual reoffending (Pithers et al., 1993; Ward and Hudson, 1998). Since then, RP has been applied to the treatment and supervision of children and adolescents with sexual behavior problems (Gray and Pithers, 1993) as well as other forms of assaultive behaviors (Cullen and Freeman-Longo, 1996).

In addition, modified relapse-prevention strategies have been found to be effective with some cognitively impaired sex offenders. Yet, as Stermac and Sheridan (1993) point out, relapse prevention emphasizes self-management and may not be appropriate for all cognitively impaired offenders. Furthermore, although interventions incorporating relapse prevention have some empirical support, few studies have investigated the specific effect of the relapse prevention efforts and results of these studies have been limited (Hanson, 1996; Marshall, 1996). Marshall has argued that current research does not justify the costs of requiring detailed training in RP concepts and extended aftercare programming for all offenders.

In addition, others (Hudson and Ward, 1996) have commented that the effectiveness of relapse prevention efforts, as perhaps with most treatment efforts, is directly related to motivation. As Gray and Pithers (1993) have noted,

A high degree of motivation and integrity is required for a client to continually monitor signs of his [or her] relapse process and to invoke coping strategies, even when it feels like a sacrifice to do so. Without the dedication derived from the empathy for sexual abuse victims developed in treatment, RP risks becoming an intellectual exercise that educates offenders about what they need to do to avoid reoffending but that finds offenders lacking the motivation to use this knowledge. (p. 299)

FACILITATING MOTIVATION
FOR POSITIVE CHANGE

Treatment compliance is important for all of the treatment areas discussed above. At a minimum, treatment compliance includes regular attendance at treatment sessions, active participation during sessions, and completion of homework assignments (Lundquist and Hansen, 1998). However, attendance alone will not assure the acquisition and maintenance of instructed parenting skills. As Dumas and Albin (1986) noted, severe adverse life circumstances such as low education, parental psychopathological symptoms, and economic stresses may impede positive outcomes.

Research and clinical experience demonstrates that poor treatment compliance is quite common among families referred for child maltreatment. Poor session attendance and high dropout rates ranging from 20 percent to 70 percent have been found (Lundquist and Hansen, 1998). Warner and colleagues (2002) found 38 percent of forty-five abusing families did not show up for home appointments, 66 percent did not show up at the clinic, and 36 percent dropped out of treatment. Rivara (as cited in Schellenbach, 1998) found that only 31 percent of seventy-one physically abusive parents complied with treatment requirements and that 30 percent of those who were compliant with treatment recidivated. Problems with treatment compliance also have been noted in the areas of sexual and partner violence (Hunter and Figueredo, 1999; Rasmussen, 1999; Saunders, 1995; Schram et al., 1991).

Parents who failed to complete treatment have been found to be more likely to have had prior complaints for abuse, have been previously treated, and to live alone or with a parent (Johnson, 1988). They also appeared less motivated, as they were less likely to volunteer for a parent-toddler interaction group and availed themselves of fewer treatment opportunities.

Reasons for noncompliance vary. Although some clients may be unmotivated and uncooperative because they do not want to engage in the recommended interventions, others may experience specific difficulties that interfere with their ability to participate in treatment. As noted earlier, sometimes these difficulties involve emotional or cognitive characteristics, such as depression or shyness (Miller and Rollnick, 1991; Patterson and Chamberlain, 1994). Cultural differences, language barriers, and family attitudes also may be obstacles (Azar et al., 1995; Dumas and Albin, 1986). Difficulties with treatment compliance may be quite pragmatic, such as when financial constraints, transportation problems, lack of child care, waiting lists, or excessive geographic distance interfere (Miller and Rollnick, 1991).

Studies have varied regarding the utility of court-ordered treatment to enhance treatment compliance in maltreating families. Wolfe and colleagues (1980) found that 74 percent of the successful outcomes were court ordered. In contrast, Irueste-Montes and Montes (1988) found that families in voluntary and court-ordered treatment participated in a comprehensive child abuse and neglect treatment program at comparable levels; however, they noted the "voluntary" clients were involved with a child protection agency and although their participation may not have been legally mandated, it also was not truly voluntary. Warner and colleagues (as cited in Lundquist and Hansen, 1998) found that court involvement was positively related to session attendance in the clinic, but not to sessions in the home. This finding suggests that the extra effort needed to attend sessions outside of the home may be facilitated by the presence of a court order.

As noted in Chapter 3, the assessment of an individual's motivation for change is important for child maltreatment interventions (Gelles, 1996), sex offender treatment (Kear-Colwell and Pollock, 1997), and partner abuse interventions (Dutton, 1996; Gondolf, 1987). For example, Gondolf suggested that Kohlberg's six stages of moral development could be utilized to facilitate the treatment of men who abuse their partners.

Using Kohlberg's developmental theory to describe men who are abusive and who are at different stages of treatment progress, Gondolf delineated three developmental levels with two stages per level. According to this theory, during the first stage of Level I, the individual is self-focused and sees others as objects to manipulate and control. The person does not perceive any wrongdoing. During the second stage of Level I, the individual begins to consider that the abusive behavior may have negative consequences but primarily is concerned with the personal impact of the consequences. If the person progresses through the developmental stages, Behavior Change (Level II) begins as the person starts to control his or her abusive behavior and subsequently becomes less emotionally isolated and more aware of the feelings of others. Further progression leads to Level III, Personal Transformation. During this stage, the individual becomes interested not only in bettering himself but also helping others and begins to live by a set of ethical principles and moral values. Gondolf argued that to be effective interventions must be tailored to the individual's level and stage of reasoning and moral development. This theory may be useful for facilitating treatment with parents who have maltreated their children.

Newman (1994) has asserted that practitioners have the obligation to understand and address client resistance in treatment and recommended specific strategies for doing so. These strategies included conducting an individualized assessment of each client's resistance by investigating the possible functions of the resistant behaviors, beliefs the individual has that may fuel the resistance, possible fears about complying with treatment, the lacking but necessary skills that could facilitate participation, the environmental factors that interfere with treatment compliance, and so forth. Once factors that contribute to the client's resistance are identified, interventions to reduce these impediments can be implemented and techniques to motivate the client, such as motivational interviewing (Miller and Rollnick, 1991) and similar approaches (Griffiths et al., 1989; Newman, 1994) can be employed. In addition, family members and significant others can be involved in treatment efforts to enhance motivation and support positive change (Egeland et al., 2000).

FINAL REMARKS

Although far from complete, the emerging research on interventions for various forms of maltreatment indicates that effective interventions are possible. The challenge remains, however, to keep refining our understanding of the optimal fit between person, problem, program, and provider.

Chapter 5

Putting It All Together

CHILD MALTREATMENT RISK ASSESSMENTS: A SPECIALIZED EVALUATION AREA

Child maltreatment risk assessments are complex, specialized evaluations. The stakes can be extremely high, involving the risk of injury or even death on the one hand, and the potential for permanent legal termination of all parent-child contact on the other. Because of the weighty nature of these issues, the legal standard imposed upon the state to justify intervention is great. Unlike divorce cases, where the issue is how skilled a parent is, in child maltreatment cases the questions focus on whether a parent is so "egregiously flawed" that state intervention is required (Dyer, 1999, p. 36) and, in the case of termination hearings, whether "there are compelling reasons to end that parent's legal right to any involvement with the child" (p. 36). Evaluators who seek to provide useful data to the courts in such complex, high-stakes cases must be familiar with the relevant literature, appropriately trained, technically skilled, and professionally competent.

A number of required core areas of knowledge have been identified (American Psychological Association Committee on Professional Practice and Standards, 1998; Dyer, 1999; Kuehnle, 1996). The areas include child, adult, and family development and behavior; parenting approaches and techniques; and individual and family dysfunction. Other necessary areas of knowledge include the effects of child maltreatment; issues pertaining to attachment, separation, and loss from primary attachment figures; and the importance of individual and cultural differences. Evaluators who assess children also should be well grounded in developmental psychopathology and the differential manifestation of certain disorders, such as dissociation

(Pearce and Pezzot-Pearce, 1997), in children as compared with adults.

Special issues when children are the subjects of assessment include research and practice findings regarding their cognitive abilities, language, memory development, and suggestibility (Kuehnle, 1996; Poole and Lamb, 1998). For example, Poole and Lamb observed that for children to be accurate informants they must first attend to the important aspects of the event in question and, subsequently, to the interviewer's directions and questions. In addition, "they must be motivated to talk and be informative, they must understand what adults are asking them, and their own memories must be protected from potentially distorting information" (p. x).

Evaluators also must be familiar with the cognitive biases and limitations in human judgment that can inadvertently impair observations and conclusions; these are discussed later in this chapter. Whether interviewing parents or children, interview techniques that are cognitively and developmentally appropriate and that attempt to avoid potential distortions by the interviewer or interviewee are needed. Various texts (e.g., Ceci and Hembrooke, 1998; Kuehnle, 1996; Poole and Lamb, 1998) are excellent sources for information about many of these issues.

Evaluators must be very circumspect about the methods they use and the conclusions they make when conducting child maltreatment evaluations. Azar and colleagues (1998) recommend "*extreme caution* in conducting such evaluations due to limitations of our current technology and the potential for biases to enter reports" (p. 78). They noted that, at present, our knowledge of what is minimally adequate parenting is unknown, tests and measures to assess questions relevant to issues of parenting abilities and child maltreatment are limited, and that there has been little study of the relationship between parental competence and children's needs, particularly among culturally, racially, and economically diverse populations.

It is essential that evaluators be fully cognizant of these limitations and keep current with the evolving professional literature. Furthermore, because we do not have assessment tools, tests, and approaches that are uniquely robust in this area, it is essential that evaluators understand that their varied methods must be used for generating hypotheses, and that they must search for convergent and divergent data through their multiple sources of information.

While recognizing the limitations of our approaches and appropriately "informing the courts as to the level of empirical foundation for findings given" (Azar et al., 1998, p. 94), child maltreatment evaluations can provide the courts with specialized knowledge that is relevant and useful for their legal determinations. As Azar and colleagues asserted, forensic mental health evaluators can use their assessment skills to gather a range of information that describes a child's developmental needs and special needs, if present, and discusses issues relevant to the parent's ability to adequately meet these needs. The provision of such information enables "more informed decisions and ones less based on emotional reactions" (p. 95).

In addition, child maltreatment risk assessments are specialized assessments because they are forensic referrals that typically involve some request for an estimation of future risk of harm or violence. As a result, evaluators must also be educated in ethical forensic practices (Perrin and Sales, 1994) and particularly in the concepts and methodology of risk assessment (Monahan, 1993) and the professional limitations regarding the prediction of violent behavior.

The disciplines of psychology and psychiatry have developed ethical guidelines pertaining both to general forensic work (American Academy of Psychiatry and the Law, 1995; Committee on Ethical Guidelines for Forensic Psychologists, 1991) and to the specialized area of child maltreatment. The specialized guidelines include the American Psychological Association's recent publication, *Guidelines for Psychological Evaluations in Child Protection Matters* (American Psychological Association Committee on Professional Practice and Standards, 1998) and the American Academy of Child and Adolescent Psychiatry's "Practice Parameters for Forensic Evaluations Involving Children and Adolescents Who May Have Been Physically or Sexually Abused" (American Academy of Child and Adolescent Psychiatry, 1997).

Interdisciplinary associations also have developed professional practice guidelines for use in child maltreatment cases. These guidelines include those published by the American Professional Society on the Abuse of Children (1995a,b, 1997) and the Association for the Treatment of Sexual Abusers (2001).

In addition to ethical codes and guidelines, evaluators also need to be familiar with relevant laws and legal procedures. For example, as noted earlier, the passage of the Adoption and Safe Families Act of

1997 requires states to expedite termination of parental rights hearings according to specified time frames so that children do not remain in temporary care for long periods of time. Expedited proceedings require evaluators to respond more quickly to evaluation requests and to complete assessments in a timely fashion.

Forensic evaluators also should be familiar with the rules of evidence that govern the types of information that can be admitted in legal proceedings and be prepared to explain their procedures, as well as their findings, to the court within this context. Review of relevant court cases, such as *Frye v. United States* (1923) and *Daubert v. Merrell-Dow Pharmaceuticals* (1993), and current legal practices relevant for child maltreatment risk assessments are available elsewhere (Dyer, 1999; Melton et al., 1997; Stern, 1997). It is of the utmost importance that forensic evaluators appreciate the legal context in which they practice and limit their interpretations and findings to statements that rest on professionally accepted procedures and methods that are validated through external sources of support.

FORENSIC VERSUS CLINICAL EVALUATIONS

Forensic evaluations differ from clinical evaluations in significant ways. A number of texts are available for a full discussion of these differences (e.g., Ackerman, 1999; Melton et al., 1997).

Briefly, in contrast to clinical evaluations, where the primary objective typically involves designing a treatment plan for a client who is experiencing psychological distress, forensic evaluations occur in response to legal questions, such as whether the risk of child maltreatment is sufficient to warrant removing a child from parental custody. As such, the primary objective of forensic evaluations is providing relevant information to a legal decision maker responsible for addressing the legal question.

The court is responsible for ultimate decisions in legal matters. However, in addition to the court, forensic evaluations may be requested by state or federal agency representatives, attorneys, and guardians (guardian ad litems), who may be appointed by the court to represent the best interests of the child (American Psychological Association Committee on Professional Practice and Standards, 1998). In order to assist the referral sources as they attempt to address the legal questions before them, forensic evaluations provide relevant objective information and unbiased conclusions and recommendations.

In contrast to clinical evaluations, where the subject of the evaluation is also the client, in a forensic evaluation the subject of the evaluation (e.g., the parent) is not the evaluator's client; the referral source, often the court, is the client. Also in contrast to clinical evaluations, where the best interests of the subject/client are paramount, in forensic evaluations, the best interests of the subject are not the central focus and, as such, findings may or may not be consistent with individual desires or therapeutic goals. In child maltreatment cases, child safety and the best interests of the child are the primary concern (American Psychological Association Committee on Professional Practice and Standards, 1998) and parental interests and rights are secondary.

When a parent has been referred for a child maltreatment risk assessment, the risks of participating in the evaluations may be perceived by the parent as many, while the benefits may be seen as few, if any. The assessment can have severe ramifications, ranging from perceived violations of privacy, as may occur from the assessment itself or from recommended service plans such as in-home interventions, to termination of parental rights. In cases involving criminal prosecution of child maltreatment, the possible consequences may include criminal convictions and incarceration for varying lengths of time. Although there may, in some cases, be benefits to parents from participating in these evaluations, such as finding mutually beneficial ways to parent their child that enhance child safety and development as well as the parent-child relationship, evaluators must recognize that these evaluations typically occur in the atmosphere of strong emotion and legitimately conflicting interests and have the potential for significant, real-world consequences. As a result, it is of the utmost importance that forensic evaluators be thorough, objective, cautious, and conservative in their practice (American Psychological Association Committee on Professional Practice and Standards, 1998).

One of the most important aspects of being cautious and thorough in conducting forensic evaluations is the recognition that, because of the stakes involved, parents, children, and others who participate in these evaluations may be intentionally or unintentionally inaccurate in their presentations. Forensic assessments may guard against these potential distortions to some degree by using multiple methods and

---

Disclosure Statement and Informed Consent

- The nature and purpose of evaluation

- Who has retained the evaluator and who owns the report

- The nonconfidential nature of evaluation

- How and to whom the evaluation report will be distributed

- The possibility of courtroom testimony

- The person being evaluated may stop the evaluation at any time to consult with counsel or to end participation until such time as he or she has had an opportunity to have his or her objection to the evaluation addressed by the legal system

---

collecting data from multiple sources, settings, and times (American Psychological Association Committee on Professional Practice and Standards, 1998).

While some have expressed concern that utilizing collateral data sources may predispose forensic evaluators to bias, the benefits of reviewing such information, as Kuehnle (1998) pointed out, typically exceed the risks because "[i]nformation from collateral sources does not stand alone but is compared and integrated with other data" (p. 4). The findings that are most reliable and warrant the greatest confidence are those that occur across situations and circumstances (Pearce and Pezzot-Pearce, 1997). As Kuehnle (1998) further noted, "If the evaluator does not collect a full spectrum of information, he or she is at risk to form less valid conclusions based on inadequate information" (p. 4).

Forensic evaluators also must be aware of their own predilections and biases. One of the ways such awareness is accomplished is by testing multiple hypotheses (Committee on Ethical Guidelines for Forensic Psychologists, 1991; Everson and Faller as cited in Kuehnle, 1998) and by evaluating data that is both consistent as well as inconsistent with the hypotheses (Borum et al., 1993). This topic is discussed in more depth later in this chapter.

In sum, the potentially severe and permanent consequences of child maltreatment risk assessments cannot be overemphasized.

Evaluators must be very conservative in their data interpretation, point out the limitations of their data, note any missing or contradictory information, and provide balanced reports that describe individual and family strengths as well as weaknesses. "It is important to attend to professional standards, ethical principles, and available research findings to guide one's evaluation. The conclusions that the practitioner draws should follow from the methodology used, and they should not extend beyond the data available" (McCann, 1998, p. 212).

COMPONENTS OF THE EVALUATION REPORT

A recent study (Budd et al., 2001) of clinical evaluations used in child protective proceedings found that parent evaluations frequently lacked information relevant to the legal issues of concern. For example, discussions of the relationship between parents' personal characteristics and behaviors and their child-rearing skills and methods often were absent. Similarly, topics such as the parents' relationships with their children frequently were lacking. In addition, evaluations often did not reflect recommended forensic practices such as clarifying and addressing referral questions, discussing the purpose of the assessment and limits of confidentiality, employing multiple methods and sources of information, using relevant tests and procedures, and so forth.

This section is offered to further assist evaluators in applying their knowledge of factors and issues relevant for child maltreatment assessment and intervention in a manner that may be most useful for referral sources.

Reason for Referral

Clinical child maltreatment risk assessments may be requested at most any stage in the child protective process. Legal issues include the need for temporary custody of the child, the appropriateness of reunification, or the necessity of termination of parental rights. The *Guidelines for Psychological Evaluations in Child Protective Matters* (American Psychological Association Committee on Professional Practice and Standards, 1998) noted that referral questions in child maltreatment cases frequently involve such questions as the following:

1. How seriously has the child's psychological well-being been affected?
2. What therapeutic interventions would be recommended to assist the child?
3. Can the parent(s) be successfully treated to prevent harm to the child in the future? If so, how? If not, why not?
4. What would be the psychological effect upon the child if returned to the parent(s)?
5. What would be the psychological effect upon the child if separated from the parents or if parental rights are terminated? (p. 4)

As noted above, the guidelines emphasize that the child's best interests and well-being are paramount in child protection evaluations.

Barnum (1997) suggested that consultation in child abuse and neglect cases involve four core issues:

1. Determining the history of abuse or neglect
2. Assessing the resulting harm to the child
3. Assessing a parent's current capacity to provide adequate care for a child
4. Predicting future risk and treatment response for children and parents

Barnum also provided a simple mnemonic to help evaluators recall these issues in consultation cases. He called the mnemonic "the four H's of child abuse" (p. 583). They are as follows:

1. What *happened?*
2. What *harm* resulted?
3. What *help* can the parents provide now?
4. What *hope* is there for the future?

Investigative interviewing designed to determine whether abuse or neglect has occurred is not the focus of this guide. However, information about what occurred is crucial to child maltreatment risk assessments. This information is important for assessing the risk of repeated incidents of maltreatment as well as for assessing possible negative effects and trauma. Further, evaluators also must recognize that the extent of past maltreatment may not be fully known at the time of referral and that appropriate forensic interviewing techniques are required (Kuehnle, 1996; Poole and Lamb, 1998).

The remaining three issues discussed by Barnum (1997)—the harm done, the parent's current capacity to safely and adequately parent the child, and the issue of prognosis—are also key components of child maltreatment risk assessments. By assessing these areas the evaluator can address questions that are central to child protective decision making. These questions can be distilled to a few, but crucial inquiries:

1. What factors increase the risk of child maltreatment?
2. What factors decrease the risk of child maltreatment?
3. What risk management plans or strategies, if any, could be used to reduce the risk of child maltreatment by ameliorating risk factors and increasing protective factors?
4. What is the parent's current and future ability to safely meet the child's developmental needs and special needs, if present?

Sometimes the parent's problems and risk factors may be so severe that an evaluation of the child is unnecessary (Dyer, 1999). More typically, however, an evaluation of the child is needed to adequately assess the child's needs and the parent's ability to safely and satisfactorily meet these needs.

In child-focused child maltreatment evaluations, the primary evaluation questions include the following:

1. What are the child's current developmental needs and special needs, if present?
2. What is the child's attachment profile? (Dyer, 1999)
3. What has been the impact of the maltreatment?
4. What interventions, if any, are required to ensure the child's safety and promote the child's healthy development?

Referral sources also may have case-specific questions that they want answered by the evaluation. These questions may help focus the evaluation and enable the evaluator to be responsive to the current concerns and issues. However, the bottom line in child maltreatment evaluations, and the only reason the state has a right to intervene in parent-child relationships, is whether a parent's actions or inaction poses a risk to a child's safety and welfare. This is the core issue that guides these important forensic evaluations.

Methods of Assessment

Disclosure Statement and Informed Consent

Parents must be made fully aware of the nature and purpose of the assessment and the risks and benefits that may be associated with the forensic child maltreatment risk assessment (American Psychological Association Committee on Professional Practice and Standards, 1998). A full disclosure of the limits or lack of confidentiality is required and should include how and to whom the evaluation report will be distributed and that the evaluator may be required to testify in court. Participants also should be informed that anything that they say may be included in the evaluation report and may be used against them in legal proceedings (Dyer, 1999).

An issue related to informed consent and the limits of confidentiality is who owns the report and who may have access to it. For example, if the referral source is the parent's attorney, the subject of the evaluation should be informed as to whether the information resulting from the assessment will be privileged (not subject to disclosure) and will be disclosed only if the attorney and the person so choose. Similarly, if the referral source is the child protective agency or the court, the subject of the evaluation should be informed that the evaluation report will be distributed to these referral sources and that the evaluation will be considered the property of the referral sources and may be disclosed further by the referral source in accordance with existing laws.

Children also should be informed, in ways consistent with the child's developmental and cognitive abilities, about why the evaluation has been requested and what it will entail. The child should be told that his or her safety is of prime importance and, because of this concern, information resulting from the assessment will be provided to others (American Psychological Association Committee on Professional Practice and Standards, 1998).

Individuals referred for child maltreatment forensic evaluations are likely to feel they have little choice but to subject themselves to the assessment process. In addition to being fully informed of the nature, purpose, and implications of participating in the evaluation, they should be told that the evaluator is not an enforcement agent for the court or other referral source. In other words, the evaluator will not insist upon their cooperation, and the individual may stop the evaluation at any time in order to confer with his or her attorney or to end his or her participation in the evaluation process. Individuals also should be informed that if they elect to refuse or terminate the evaluation, this information will be provided to the referral source and the subject, in conjunction with his or her attorney, will then have the opportunity to discuss and resolve this issue with the referral source. If the subject then returns to complete the evaluation, or is ordered to do so, the evaluator should not view the individual's exercise of his or her legal rights with prejudice.

Informed consent must be obtained before proceeding with the evaluation. Some states require written consent (American Psychological Association Committee on Professional Practice and Standards, 1998) and this seems advisable regardless of statutory differences.

Sources of Information

As described in Chapters 2 and 3, various factors contribute to increase the risk and negative effects of maltreatment. As previously noted, multiple methods and sources of information are required to enhance accuracy and to facilitate appropriate conclusions and recommendations. It is important that evaluators be active in requesting relevant information, and not be passive (Saunders, 1997), simply relying on what is provided. It also is important that evaluators be alert to possible biases and distortions that may exist in the information provided (Azar et al., 1998). As noted in the Professional Issues discussion later in this chapter, in addition to the possibility of intentional distortions, errors in information processing, human judgment, and decision making may contribute to inaccuracies in the information received (e.g., Borum et al., 1993; Poole and Lamb, 1998).

Maltreating parents and individuals typically underreport their abusive behavior (Saunders, 1995) and attempt to present themselves in the best possible light (Quinsey et al., 1996). When conducting forensic evaluations it may be possible to find common goals with the subject of the evaluation that will facilitate the assessment process. More often, however, resistance, minimizing, and denial are common impediments to the evaluation task.

In order to offset these problems, evaluations should, where feasible, include a review of relevant records, collateral contacts, clinical interviews, mental status examinations, behavioral observations, and relevant psychological testing. Recent reports documenting why the issue of maltreatment has surfaced at this time obviously are important sources of information, as are historical and legal documents that provide information about the possibility of previous instances of maltreatment. Unless the child's needs have been evaluated separately, the child should be interviewed or assessed. Whenever possible and if it is safe for the child, the parent and child should be observed together (Azar et al., 1998; Dyer, 1999; Melton et al., 1997).

Sources of information may be direct, such as self-reports and behavioral observations. Multiple sessions under varying levels of stress provide a greater sampling of behaviors and have been recommended (Azar et al., 1998; Budd et al., 2001).

Indirect sources of information include child protective service records and police records, reports from treatment providers, foster parent interviews, and interviews with family members and significant others who are not the focus of the evaluations. The following list includes possible sources of information.

- Self-report (clinical interview and mental status examination)
- Behavioral observations
- Parent-child observation
- Psychological testing
- Child protective agency records and reports (in-state and out of state)
- Federal, state, and local police investigative reports, pictures, and audio and video tapes
- Arrests and conviction records
- Probation and parole records
- District attorney records
- Defense attorney reports
- Victim witness advocate and guardian ad litem reports

- Foster parent interviews and reports
- Treatment records and prior evaluations (mental health and medical)
- Substance abuse records
- Relevant family member evaluations
- Reports from family members and significant others
- School, work, and military records
- Previous victim interview reports, medical and/or mental health reports
- Interviews with family, friends, employers, and significant others

As Saunders (1997) recommended, evaluators should carefully review primary documents and not simply rely on secondary reports. Whenever possible, background information should be reviewed before interviews are conducted so that the evaluator has a good understanding of the history and issues involved in the case (Dyer, 1999).

When reporting information it is important to attribute information to its source. If unverified information is used in the report, its uncorroborated nature must be apparent. Information about whether the individual agrees or disagrees with the allegations also should be provided. Disagreements should not be clinically described as denial or as untrue unless the veracity of the underlying allegations has been clearly determined. Statements relating to allegations that have not been proven should always be presented in a way that clearly reflects their hypothetical nature. For example, "These allegations, if true, would be seen as consistent (or inconsistent) with the clinical data which suggests . . ." or "If these allegations are true, treatment should include . . ."

Structured and Focused Clinical Interviews

Clinical interviews serve multiple functions. These functions include obtaining informed consent, establishing adequate rapport, providing the opportunity for observations of behaviors and attitudes, and gathering information about the individual's perceptions of his or her history and involvement with the child protective agency (Dyer, 1999). Interviews with children may assist evaluators in assessing the precipitants for maltreatment, evaluating the nature and strength of the parent-child relationship, and assessing each child's needs for treatment or intervention and whether the children have suffered negative effects as a result of their maltreatment. In addition, conjoint interviews with parents, child-parent interviews, and family interviews may provide further useful information.

Research studies, however, have found that clinical judgment and decision making can be negatively affected by a range of cognitive biases and information-processing errors (Poole and Lamb, 1998). Evaluation protocols and structured interviews may help reduce some of these problems; for example, by requiring evaluators to probe areas they may otherwise have missed (Poole and Lamb, 1998). Risk assessment protocols, such as those discussed later in this chapter, can be used to structure and enhance interviews. Interviews that are overly structured may suppress, however, evidence of some types of psychopathology (Hare, 1991). Inquiries related to child developmental histories and trauma also may be facilitated by structured interviews and guides such as those presented by Pearce and Pezzot-Pearce (1997). In addition, this guide summarizes the professional literature in ways that are designed to guide and facilitate child maltreatment evaluations.

As noted earlier, several texts (e.g., Kuehnle, 1996; Poole and Lamb, 1998) are excellent sources for information on conducting developmentally sensitive interviews with children. Poole and Lamb, for example, reviewed findings concerning the effectiveness of various interviewing approaches. They also provided interview guidelines that were distilled from several sources which may enhance the accuracy of children's reports. These recommendations included that children be interviewed as soon as possible after alleged events. The guidelines also suggest that children should be provided with sufficient time "to acclimate to the interviewing environment, build rapport with the interviewer, receive instructions about the 'rules' of the interview (e.g., their right to say 'no' or to ask for clarification of a question), and practice being informative" (p. 72).

In addition, Poole and Lamb noted that open-ended questions are primary. When focused questions are required to clarify information they should be presented in ways that maximize response options and then should be followed by more open-ended or general questions. In addition to maintaining a neutral stance, evaluators are encouraged to consider multiple interpretations of the child's statements. When completing interviews, depending upon the child's age and circumstances, opportunities to review and clarify what the child reported should be provided, as well as information about how the evaluator can be contacted after the evaluation. The interview should close after a discussion of more neutral topics spoken in a supportive manner. Poole and Lamb noted that, for the most part, research findings have not supported the use of ancillary aids (such as drawings and anatomically correct dolls). The authors remarked, "As with most forensic and investigative protocols, we take a conservative approach and recommend that interviewers focus on strategies that encourage verbal reports, using interview aids sparingly and cautiously, if at all" (p. 203).

As noted earlier in this chapter, forensic evaluations involve a range of issues that are not typically present in most clinical settings. For example, the possibility of impression-management response styles must be assessed (McCann and Dyer, 1996). Evaluators should also be sensitive to the likelihood that many adults and children involved in child maltreatment assessments may be experiencing anxiety, embarrassment, feelings of shame and guilt, and may feel stigmatized (Pearce and Pezzot-Pearce, 1997).

Parent-Child Observations

Observations of parent-child interactions have been described as a very important source of information (Azar et al., 1998; Dyer, 1999; Melton et al., 1997). Observations provide direct behavioral information about parent and child behaviors and may provide important information about their relationship (Dyer, 1999).

When conducting assessments, the reliability and validity of evaluation techniques must, however, always be considered. A review of the literature on parent-child interaction assessment approaches (The Assessment of Parent-Child Interactions, 1998) revealed concerns about whether such techniques have adequate reliability and validity, even in nonforensic settings. Milner and colleagues (1998) reported that, similar to interviews, observational approaches often have modest reliability and validity. They noted that studies of observational approaches often have revealed group differences between abusive and nonabusive parents, but attempts to classify individual parents have had mixed results.

Because subjective judgment is required during observational assessments, various evaluator characteristics and biases may negatively affect the validity of observational assessment methods (Azar et al., 1998; Milner et al., 1998). As noted earlier, these factors are discussed in more depth later in this chapter. Because of these potential problems and difficulties, it is essential that, if evaluators use parent-child interaction observations, they use these approaches cautiously, with awareness of the strengths and limitations of these evaluation methods, and in conjunction with alternative measures and collateral sources.

With the above cautions in mind, parent-child observations can be conducted in the home or office. Activities should be age appropriate, realistic, and reflective of relevant behaviors and issues, such as disciplinary styles (Milner et al., 1998). Activities may include feeding, structured tasks, free play, and separation and reunion (Clark, 1985). With older children activities may include a teaching task, cooperative activities, a problem-solving task, and clean up (Schutz et al., 1989). Qualitative factors, such as the frequency and kinds of touching, eye contact and smiles, a child's comfort and guidance seeking behaviors, and the parent's responsiveness to the child's expressed needs may reflect important aspects of the parent-child relationship (Sasserath et al. as cited in Dyer, 1999).

Some observational approaches are very structured, requiring extensive training and, sometimes, certification that the "researcher" conducting the assessment has demonstrated adequate inter-rater reliability (Solomon and George, 1999). There are a number of structured observational approaches available, particularly for younger children, that are reviewed elsewhere (e.g., Azar et al., 1998; Mash, 1991; Solomon and George, 1999). However, as Azar and colleagues noted, standardized norms for rating interactions, especially in situations where a child may have spent significant time separated from the parent, and predictive validity data pertaining to child maltreatment outcomes are currently lacking. Therefore, when such approaches are used as part of a child maltreatment evaluation, caution is advised.

Smith (1991) noted that observational approaches are always subject to the question whether the behaviors observed are characteristic of the subjects or whether they are in response to the observation. He suggested that the validity of these approaches can be enhanced by the evaluator being as unobtrusive as possible, establishing good rapport, and allowing the evaluation participants to become acclimated to the evaluation situation. Others (Sasserath et al. as cited in Dyer, 1999), however, have argued that attachment cannot be faked and that observational assessments will be able to distinguish between behaviors and emotions in the child that have been reinforced over time in contrast to immediate reaction to evaluation-specific parental behaviors. Such arguments, however, have not been empirically demonstrated, and thus this issue remains open.

Home-based observations may be more ecologically valid than office-based assessments, but they too are vulnerable to impression management. Furthermore, home observations are time intensive and may not be economically possible. In either case, clearly abusive or neglectful behavior during a parent-child assessment would be revealing, but other behaviors may be more difficult to assess.

When termination of parental rights issues are involved, parent-child observations of the child with the foster or preadoptive parents as well as the birth parents are thought to facilitate the evaluation of the child's primary attachment (Dyer, 1999). When observations with the birth parents are strongly resisted by the child, experienced by the child as harmful, in any way place the child in jeopardy, or have been legally prohibited, they are contraindicated (American Psychological Association Committee on Professional Practice and Standards, 1998; Dyer, 1999).

Psychometric Testing

Psychological tests that are relevant to the referral questions can provide valuable risk assessment and management information. Relevant psychological tests may include personality measures, abuse-specific assessment instruments, measures of cognitive functioning and, possibly, psychophysiological techniques. The utility and appropriate use of various adult- and child-focused instruments that may be appropriate for child maltreatment risk assessments have been reviewed elsewhere and will not be detailed here (Dyer, 1999; Heinze and Grisso, 1996; Kuehnle, 1996; Milner and Murphy, 1995; Milner et al., 1998).

Whenever tests and measures are used in child maltreatment risk assessments, they must be used appropriately. Heilbrun (1992) provided guidelines to assist forensic evaluators in selecting psychological tests. He emphasized that psychological tests used in forensic settings should have acceptable levels of reliability and validity and be relevant to referral questions. His recommendations also included such issues as whether the test is commercially available and adequately documented by a test manual and an additional source. Other guidelines address the standardization of test administration and the applicability of a test for a given individual and purpose, as well as the preference for objective tests and actuarial procedures when appropriate outcome data are available and an empirically based assessment procedure or formula exists. The guidelines also addressed the issue of assessing individual respondents' test response styles and using such findings when interpreting test results. Although Heilbrun's guidelines have been described as very conservative (Ackerman, 1999), they can help guide evaluators in appropriate test selection and assist them in preparing for possible challenges pertaining to the tests they select.

Because impression management and defensive responding during forensic evaluations commonly occur, test instruments that evaluate such issues may be particularly useful (Borum et al., 1993). It is important to remember, however, that no psychological test, instrument, or clinical interview can determine whether child maltreatment or interpersonal violence has, in fact, occurred. Although some perpetrators of child maltreatment and interpersonal violence share some characteristics, they are heterogeneous and there is no singular offender profile. More specific to the issue of psychological testing is Milner and Murphy's (1995) review of interview and observational techniques, psychological assessment instruments, and measures of psychophysiological reactivity used in child physical and sexual abuse evaluations, and their conclusions. They reported that

> A review of the literature related to the use of general assessment measures with child physical and sexual abusers indicates that there is no one profile and no single characteristic that has been consistently found in these rather heterogeneous populations . . . . Nevertheless, the use of general assessment procedures may have some value in treatment planning. For example, extant standardized measures may identify significant areas of dysfunction in the offender . . . that are in need of remediation, but this should not be confused with suggestions that these fac-

tors have some type of etiological significance or represent characteristics found in most child physical or sexual abusers. (p. 4)

Increasingly, there have been attempts to develop specialized assessment techniques that relate specifically to questions about parents' current and future parenting abilities (Heinze and Grisso, 1996). Examples of these assessment instruments include the Child Abuse Potential Inventory (CAP) (Milner, 1986) and the Parent Stress Inventory (Abidin, 1995).

The CAP is a psychometric instrument that assesses the extent to which an individual's pattern of responses is similar to those of individuals who are known to have physically abused their children. CAP items reflect attitudes, traits, and behaviors that are empirically associated with child physical abuse. Higher scores on the CAP inventory are associated with increased risk for physical child abuse. Although the psychometric properties of the CAP inventory have been described as strong, they may result in false positive classifications among emotionally distressed or mentally ill parents, or parents of children who are handicapped, learning disabled, or physically ill (Heinze and Grisso, 1996). Further, because of the probabilistic nature of test scores, elevated scores can never be used to confirm whether or not specific acts of abuse have occurred or will occur.

PSI was developed as a screening instrument to assess the level of stress that a parent is experiencing in the child-rearing role (Heinze and Grisso, 1996). The PSI provides a total stress score as well as subscales that measure stress in the child domain and the parent domain. An optional set of questions composes the life stress domain and assesses major stresses that have occurred during the past year.

Heinze and Grisso (1996) reported that the psychometric properties of the PSI are very strong, but they urged caution in interpreting findings. High scores cannot be interpreted as indicators of the presence or absence of child maltreatment, or that a parent is unable to parent adequately. Rather, high scores should be interpreted to suggest that high levels of child-rearing related stress may be present and that the possibility of dysfunctional parenting behaviors, or possible problem behaviors in the child, should be carefully considered. Low scores may reflect low levels of parenting-related stress but also may reflect defensive responding, a neglectful parent, or a parent who is not very invested in parenting (Heinze and Grisso, 1996).

The Multiphasic Sex Inventory (MSI) (Nichols and Molinder, 1984) is an instrument that was designed to describe relevant psychosexual characteristics of male sex offenders. Reviewers described the MSI as having clinical utility for descriptive purposes in populations of known sex offenders (Milner and Murphy, 1995). The MSI also was described as providing incremental information beyond standard psychological instruments (Kalichman et al., 1992). However, empirical investigations of the MSI and its validity have been described as limited (Bourke and Donohue, 1996; Milner and Murphy, 1995). The Multiphasic Sex Inventory-II (MSI-II) (Nichols and Molinder, 1996) is a revision of the MSI. Published, peer-reviewed reports on the psychometric properties of the MSI-II do not appear available at this time.

The Hare Psychopathy Checklist – Revised (Hare, 1991) (PCL-R) measures the extent to which the subject matches the profile of the prototypic psychopath. Research studies (e.g., Harris et al., 1993; Quinsey et al., 1995; Salekin et al., 1996; Serin, 1996) have demonstrated that psychopathy, as measured by the PCL-R, is a strong predictor of violent behavior in general and sexual violence among adult offenders (Quinsey et al., 1995; Serin et al., 1994), as well as juvenile delinquency (Forth et al., 1990; Hare, 1991). Although relatively small proportions of sex offenders have been found to be psychopathic (Serin et al., 1994), diagnoses of psychopathy and phallometrically assessed sexual interest in nonsexual violence toward women have been found to be as predictive of new sexual offenses and other kinds of violent offenses by adult male rapists as were predictions made from a greater number of predictors (Rice et al., 1990).

In addition, the literature shows that not only do psychopaths begin their criminal careers earlier than other offenders, they commit more types of offenses, and perpetrate a disproportionate number of violent acts during their incarceration or hospitalization (Forth et al., 1990; Hare, 1991; Hare et al., 1988; and Serin, 1996). Psychopathic individuals as measured by the PCL-R have been found to have higher rates of recidivism on conditional release and post discharge (Forth et al., 1990; Hart et al., 1988; Serin et al., 1990; Harris et al., 1993). They recidivate sooner, offend at a higher rate than nonpsychopaths, and are more likely to reoffend violently (Harris et al., 1991; Hart et al., 1988).

Gacono and Hutton (1994) described referral indicators for a PCL-R assessment as including cases of suspected malingering, treatment amenability, lengthy criminal histories, antisocial personality disorder diagnoses, histories of predatory violence, violence potential, and correctional decisions involving outpatient placement, parole, and classification. The utility of the PCL-R in assessing a parent's ability to adequately parent their child in safe and nonmaltreating ways does not appear to have been empirically investigated. However, characteristics of psychopathic individuals, such as egocentricity; impulsivity; irresponsibility; shallow emotions; lack of empathy, guilt, and remorse; manipulating; persistent violation of social norms; and so forth (Hare, 1996) are generally inconsistent with adequately providing for a child's developmental needs. When parental histories are consistent with the PCL-R normative populations (i.e., criminal or forensic psychiatric groups), the PCL-R may provide useful information. Yet, as Gacono and Hutton (1994) noted, "The PCL-R provides access to one variable—psychopathy level—whereas most clinical questions require multiple methods (battery) to provide valid recommendations. Often a combination of structured and unstructured assessment tools such as the PCL-R, record review, Rorschach test, and the MMPI, along with an assessment of cognitive functioning, can address most forensic referral questions" (p. 309).

As previously noted, parental assessments in child maltreatment cases focus on the "nexus . . . between the individual's psychopathology and specific deficiencies in parenting capacity" (Dyer, 1999, p. 99). Thus, related assessment procedures may include measures of intellectual and cognitive functioning, personality and psychological functioning, and psychopathology. Psychological testing also may be useful for assessing specific attitudes, values, beliefs, and other psychological factors pertaining to child abuse and neglect, sexual violence, and partner abuse. When test instruments have not been validated on the populations to which an individual is assigned (i.e., parents who have maltreated or children who have been maltreated), evaluators must use these instruments cautiously and appropriately (Melton et al., 1997).

Psychological evaluations of children who have been maltreated also may benefit from psychological tests that provide information concerning the child's developmental and personality functioning. These may include measures of cognitive and intellectual functioning as well as emotional and behavioral functioning.

Behavior rating scales may provide important normative information about the child's strengths and vulnerabilities. Scales such as the Child Behavior Checklist (CBCL) (Achenbach, 1991) cover a broad range of children's competencies and problems. However, special caution must be used when behavior rating scales or other instruments lack measures of possible response biases. Response biases can significantly distort findings. For example, researchers (Everson et al., 1989) found little concordance between the descriptions of child behaviors on the CBCL provided by mothers who provided ambivalent or minimal support to their children and the results of a structured interview conducted with the child. Conversely, there was substantial concordance between the reports of supportive mothers and their children. The authors hypothesized that, at times, a parent's perceptions of a child may be more of a reflection of the parent's personality and adjustment difficulties than an accurate picture of the child's level of functioning. Utilizing multiple informants and cross informant comparisons as well as multiple sources of information is clearly important for managing possible biases.

With this caution in mind, information about a child's adaptive behavior skills, such as self-feeding and using the toilet, basic social skills, and so forth, can be measured with an instrument such as the Vineland Adaptive Behavior Scales (Dyer, 1999; Pearce and Pezzot-Pearce, 1997). Dyer strongly recommended this form of assessment when a parent's functioning is marginal and when questions exist about how self-sufficient the child is.

Another example of relevant tests and instruments is the Child Sexual Behavior Inventory (CSBI) (Friedrich, 1997). The CSBI is a measure of sexual behavior in children as described by a child's female parent or caretaker. A wide range of sexual behavior is included. Findings from the CSBI provide data regarding the overall level of sexual behavior exhibited by the child, sexual behaviors that may be considered as normative for the child's age and gender, and sexual behaviors that may be viewed as atypical for the child's age and gender.

During the past decade there has been a widespread increase in efforts to develop instruments designed to specifically measure the impact of trauma on children (and adults). Many of these are in various states of development and differ in their psychometric maturity. Stamm (1996) has reviewed this area and provides an excellent guide to these instruments and their various properties. Some, such as The Trauma Symptom Checklist for Children (TSCC) (Briere, 1996), a psychometric test that is designed to evaluate acute and chronic post-traumatic stress and other psychological effects of traumatic events, have been commercially published and are widely available. In spite of the potential utility of abuse- and trauma-specific instruments such as the TSCC, as noted in Chapter 2, some maltreated children are asymptomatic.

Clinicians who utilize psychological tests require specialized training in administering and interpreting them and should be able to evaluate the psychometric qualities of the tests that they use. The importance of appropriate training cannot be overemphasized. Recognizing this importance, the New Jersey Board of Psychological Examiners has mandated that evaluators who utilize psychological tests and measures be able to interpret these instruments independently and not solely rely on computerized narrative reports (Dyer, 1999).

Psychophysiological Assessment

Psychophysiological assessment techniques include phallometric evaluations of sex offenders. Phallometric assessments typically are used to provide standardized measurements of sexual arousal by direct measurement of penile circumference or volume (Milner et al., 1998). This assessment procedure is used to obtain specific information regarding an individual's sexual arousal to various standardized stimuli such as age and gender preference and interest in sexual violence relative to consensual sexual interactions. The use of phallometric procedures requires special equipment and training.

Milner and colleagues (1998) summarized the strengths and limitations of this procedure and provided references for more technical reviews. They noted that the strengths of phallometric assessments include research demonstrating that groups of extrafamilial sex offenders could be reliably differentiated from nonoffenders and other offender groups. Studies also have found positive correlations between deviant sexual arousal, as measured by phallometric assessments, and recidivism that exceed associations between other risk factors and recidivism.

Other studies, however, have found less promising results (Milner et al., 1998). In contrast to groups of extrafamilial sex offenders, individual offenders have been more difficult to reliably classify. Many perpetrators of child sexual abuse do not evidence deviant arousal when assessed and some demonstrate very low levels of sexual arousal. In addition, research has shown that responses during phallometric assessments can be intentionally altered, however procedures have been developed that may reduce a respondent's ability to control his penile responses (e.g., Proulx et al., 1993). In spite of this advance, other limitations of phallometric assessments exist and include limited reliability data as well as limited information about how subject factors such as ethnicity or emotional states may affect the validity of these procedures (Milner et al., 1998).

As the above findings reflect, phallometric assessments may provide some useful clinical information in some cases. When used, their limitations must be fully considered. Assessments of deviant arousal do not reflect whether a sexual offense has occurred and never should be used in this manner.

Psychophysiological assessment procedures also have been used in research settings to evaluate the psychophysiological reactivity of people who have physically abused their children or who were considered at risk of doing so. Findings have been mixed and questions about the ecological validity of psychophysiological assessment exist (Milner et al., 1998).

Risk Assessment Protocols

The finding that actuarial predictions of a wide range of behaviors are superior to unstructured clinical determinations has persisted over many years of research (Melton et al., 1997; Steadman et al., 2000). Recent years have seen the development of various violence assessment tools that are designed to facilitate more accurate assessments of violent behavior. Some risk assessment protocols pertain to general violence, such as the Violence Risk Appraisal Guide (VRAG) (Quinsey et al., 1998) and the HCR-20 (H-historical, C-clinical, R-risk management) (Webster et al., 1997a). Other protocols are more offense specific, such as the Static-99 (Hanson and Thornton, 2000), Sex Offender Risk Appraisal Guide (SORAG) (Quinsey et al., 1998), the Sexual Violence Risk-20 (SVR-20) (Boer et al., 1997), the Spousal

Assault Risk Assessment Guide (SARA) (Kropp et al., 1995), the Juvenile Sex Offender Assessment Protocol (J-SOAP) (Prentky & Righthand, 2001), and the Estimate of Risk of Adolescent Sexual Offense Recidivism, Version 2.0 (ERASOR) (Worling & Curwen, 2000). Some of these instruments, such as the HCR-20, SVR-20, J-SOAP, ERASOR, and the SARA are checklists of empirically based variables that are associated with the targeted violent behavior. These instruments are designed to facilitate comprehensive evaluations and risk assessments by ensuring that relevant factors are assessed but are not intended to provide statistical predictions of recidivism (Borum, 1996). Other instruments, such as the VRAG and SORAG, are actuarial measures that produce estimated statistical probabilities of long-term risk. These instruments, however, rely heavily on largely historical and therefore static variables and may, consequently, be less sensitive to shorter term fluctuations in risk that are more reflective of changes in current, dynamic, and changeable risk factors. Although the available instruments advance the field of risk assessment, cross-validation research and relevant norms as well as instruments that include a wider range of dynamic variables are needed.

Risk assessment is not new to the field of child maltreatment assessment. Although reports discussing the utilization of structured or actuarial risk assessments in clinical and forensic child maltreatment evaluations appear lacking, child protective agencies have been developing formal risk assessment procedures throughout the past couple of decades (English and Marshall, 1998; Milner et al., 1998). Milner and colleagues observed that specialized child maltreatment risk assessment procedures were developed to improve risk assessment determinations by providing more consistent, structured, and systematic assessments that considered parent factors as well as child, demographic, and other case-specific variables.

Substantial variability in the risk assessment approaches used by different states and even between different agencies within states has been reported (English and Marshall, 1998; Milner, 1998). There is considerable variability in the types and number of risk factors used in child protective risk assessments as well as how the risk assessment measures are designed. Most risk assessment protocols, however, do include factors that assess the nature and chronicity of the maltreatment, the caregivers' history of child maltreatment, domestic violence, and the family's social and economic circumstances. Child characteristics and the nature of the parent-child relationship also are typically assessed. English and Marshall (1998) noted that these risk assessments

> share the common philosophy that certain factors operating in the lives of troubled families tend to increase or decrease the likelihood of child maltreatment, and proper identification and consideration of these factors can help set priorities and inform. (p. 123)

Some states have developed actuarial risk assessment instruments to identify and classify the risk of future child maltreatment that individuals or families may present (Abernathy et al., 1998; Bell and Wagner, 1998; English and Marshall, 1998). Most of these assessment instruments were developed in collaboration with the National Center for Crime and Delinquency and then adapted to conform to the individual state's laws, policies, program practices, and ongoing research (Moore, 1998). Some of the states have separate risk assessment scales for abuse and neglect that enable classifying risk levels for each type of child maltreatment (Bell and Wagner, 1998; Meyer and Wagner, 1998). Typically, these instruments also allow for the actuarial classification to be modified based on professional judgment or policy determinations (Bell and Wagner, 1998; Meyer and Wagner, 1998).

Other states use risk assessment protocols that, like actuarial instruments, are based on risk factors that have been identified by research to be associated with the risk of child maltreatment, but that typically do not base risk classifications on numerical scoring systems or composite scores (Abernathy et al., 1998). This latter type of risk assessment protocol is designed primarily to facilitate risk management decisions by helping caseworkers to systematically structure their information gathering, synthesis, and analysis (S. Hodge, personal communication, March 2000). Such risk assessment protocols "serve as heuristic devices to trigger worker memory of possible risk factors overlooked in the investigations" (Abernathy et al., 1998, p. 1).

Milner and colleagues (1998) noted that one source of problems with the current risk assessment approaches involves the inclusion of items that have been associated with child maltreatment but that have not yet been shown to be causally related to or predictive of abuse or reabuse. Another problem is that some agencies use a single risk assessment instrument that does not differentiate between cases which present with different forms of abuse or multiple types of maltreatment that may result from different constellations of risk factors. Still other problems are similar to difficulties in the areas of predicting violence in general and include a range of methodological problems that contribute to difficulties establishing the predictive validity of child maltreatment instruments, such as identifying appropriate criterion measures and base rate concerns (English and Pecora, 1994).

Child maltreatment risk assessment protocols also suffer from reliability problems. For example, Murphy-Berman (1994) pointed out that although some risk factors may be overt and obvious and, therefore, easily assessed, others may be less observable and result in more subjective assessments and reduced reliability. Other risk assessment problems include concerns about whether child protective workers are sufficiently trained in risk assessment procedures, how well they implement assessment protocols, whether such protocols are utilized in a reliable manner, and whether risk assessment findings are, even when available, actually used in decision making (DePanfilis, 1996b; Doueck and Lyons, 1998; English and Marshall, 1998).

Milner and Campbell (1995) noted that another reason why child maltreatment risk assessments may be problematic is that intervening variables can occur after the evaluation which may increase or decrease the risk of abuse. Thus, even a reliable and valid risk assessment instrument may be subject to prediction errors due to intervening variables. In some cases, this source of error may be reduced by timely decision making that occurs soon after the completion of the risk assessment and also by periodic reassessment, especially regarding dynamic risk factors that are most subject to short-term fluctuations.

Some of the problems discussed above are relevant to actuarial risk assessment in general and require thoughtful consideration. Research findings indicate that actuarial risk assessment tools are rarely utilized in daily clinical practice (Steadman et al., 2000). Various explanations of this finding have been offered (Melton et al., 1997; Steadman et al., 2000), for example, people tend to prefer case-specific information and ignore statistical data.

Melton and colleagues (1997) noted that few research studies have compared actuarial and clinical assessment approaches, and, of the few studies that did, the improvement in predictive accuracy of the actuarial approaches was only "meager." The few existing studies generally have been conducted at single sites and have involved small samples. Cross-validation research typically has been lacking and the applicability of site-specific findings to other settings is open to question. In sum, Melton and his colleagues stressed, "The bottom line is that the research has not delivered an actuarial equation suitable for clinical application in the area of violence prediction" (pp. 284-285).

Another problem with actuarial approaches is that they generally utilize linear regression models that suggest that there is one solution that is applicable for each person assessed (Steadman et al., 2000). Melton and colleagues (1997) pointed out that such actuarial techniques typically do not allow for the consideration of relevant case-specific information. Because of these concerns, these authors concluded:

> Absent a proven formula we must continue, in Meehl's words, to "use our heads." . . . By reading the published literature, clinicians can identify factors from a variety of domains (e.g., demographics and clinical features) that have established empirical correlations with violence. Depending on the features present and the strength of their associations with violence recidivism, the presence of more, or fewer, such factors in an individual case may then guide judgments about that person's relative risk for violence. (p. 285)

As Melton and colleagues (1997) pointed out, however, this recommendation does not suggest that risk assessment is as easy as adding up risk factors on a list. Although an increased number of risk factors may be associated with a greater risk of offending, in some cases the presence of even one or two may be critical (Webster et al., 1997b). Furthermore, the ways that risk, individual strengths, and other mitigating factors interact often complicate the equation and must be considered.

Assessment Domains

Child maltreatment does not occur in a vacuum (Pearce and Pezzot-Pearce, 1997). As noted in Chapters 2 and 3, child maltreatment and its effects involve many different risk factors as well as potential moderating variables that occur on various different levels and include individual, family, and community factors, as well as larger societal factors. The interactions of these factors are often quite complex and, depending on the referral questions, the domains of assessment include consideration of individual factors, the parent-child relationship, family variables, social issues (such as poverty and neighborhood quality), as well as class, cultural, and societal norms (Azar et al., 1998; Pearce and Pezzot-Pearce, 1997).

Whatever the relevant assessment domains are in an evaluation of a specific case, in essence, child maltreatment risk assessments are functional assessments. As such, they have to focus on the pragmatics of a parent's competence to parent in ways that at least minimally promote the child's safety and development (Melton et al., 1997). Functional assessment of parents require evaluation of the parent's current abilities, attitudes, and behaviors, and the likely interaction of these factors with a child's individual and developmental needs and other situational demands as they arise over time (Azar et al., 1998; Grisso, 1986; Wolfe, 1985). More specifically, as Azar and colleagues (1998) argued, child maltreatment evaluations require a "functional-contextual framework" where data "link parents' *individual skills/deficits* with their capacity to parent *a particular child* within the *specific* contexts that are available to them (e.g., quality of marriage, social supports, socioeconomic status, neighborhoods)" (p. 77).

As noted in Chapter 3, relevant assessment areas include such issues as parents' ability to accurately perceive and make appropriate attributions of their children's behaviors, to have developmentally appropriate expectations of the child, to differentiate their own needs from their child's, and to respond appropriately to the child. Other relevant issues include parents' behavior management skills, problem-solving abilities, facilitation of the child's relationships and attachments, and ability to appropriately monitor their children and protect them from harm. Furthermore, parents' motivation to make needed changes to enhance their parenting abilities and parent-child relationship is important.

Assessments of children in child maltreatment cases also focus on functional issues. These issues include the child's current level of functioning as well as the presence of risk factors associated with negative outcomes for the child, such as emotional, behavioral, and learning problems. Other relevant issues include the child's attachments to parents, foster parents, and significant others. When a child is in out-of-home placement, the age at placement and the number of placements may be important considerations (Dyer, 1999). Particular attention must be paid to any special needs or challenges that may be present and persist over time. For example, medical conditions that require vigilant parental attention and competent responses, such as severe asthma or insulin-dependent diabetes, and "impose an increased burden of care" (Dyer, 1999, p. 128) must be identified and considered.

Finally, the parent's ability to make the requisite judgments, decisions, and responses to adequately meet the child's social, emotional, cognitive, behavioral, and medical needs should be assessed. It is essential that the assessment consider not only the child's current development needs but also his or her future developmental needs (Azar et al., 1998). When reunification is a possibility it is necessary to assess the parent's ability to appropriately support the child, who may grieve the loss of his or her foster parent and family, and to respond nonpunitively and supportively to the child's behavioral and emotional responses (Dyer, 1999).

Dyer also argued that evaluations of children in child maltreatment cases require "bonding evaluations" (p. 8) that assess the nature and quality of children's attachments to their birth parents and their foster parents so as to determine who is most central to the child's life and development (p. 8). He noted that young preschool-aged children are very much engaged in the process of personality formation.

> Their day-to-day interactions with caretakers provide the raw material, as it were, for identifications, emotional connections, and attitudes that shape their sense of themselves, capacity for mood regulation, anxiety tolerance, impulse control, basic trust, self-confidence and optimism, and behavior in future intimate relationships. (p. 11)

Separations from primary attachment figures can have detrimental effects on children's development. The effects of such separations have important implications for visitation schedules and reunification when children are separated from parents. Dyer (1999) emphasized that when children have been placed in alternative care and develop primary attachments to a significant caregiver other than the parent, it is necessary to evaluate the future harm that may result from removing the child from the attachment figure. Placing such children with their biological parents may be like placing them with people who seem like strangers to the child. A more detailed review of attachment issues in child maltreatment situations and related assessment strategies is beyond the scope of this guide, but can be found elsewhere (e.g., Dyer, 1999; Pearce and Pezzot-Pearce, 1997).

When conducting child maltreatment risk assessments, a critical area of investigation that warrants special attention is the nature and context of the child maltreatment. Such analyses involve assessing the details of the maltreatment. Pearce and Pezzot-Pearce (1997) described the analysis as involving identifying the following factors:

1. The types of maltreatment
2. The age of the child when the maltreatment began
3. The frequency and duration of the maltreatment
4. The relationship of the perpetrator or perpetrators to the child
5. The extent to which the child was threatened or coerced physically or psychologically

Other relevant assessment areas include the factors that preceded the maltreatment as well as what circumstances occurred following the maltreatment. This question involves the assessment of affective states as well as behaviors. Inquiry also will involve questions about how the maltreatment was disclosed or discovered, the response of the child as well as the child protective and legal system (Pearce and Pezzot-Pearce, 1997), and the response of significant others, such as parents or other family members who have not been identified as perpetrators. A thorough analysis of the maltreating behavior and related circumstances is necessary so as to fully understand how and why the maltreatment occurred and what may be done to decrease the likelihood of such behaviors in the future.

The risk assessment format described in Chapter 3, based on the assessment domains used by MacArthur Violence Risk Assessment Study (The MacArthur Study, 2001) appears useful for guiding parent and child assessments. This format includes historical and demographic variables as well as dynamic clinical and situational variables that are associated with child maltreatment and the negative emotional and behavioral outcomes that may be associated with the maltreatment. The assessment areas include the following:

1. Historical or developmental factors
2. Dispositional or personal factors
3. Clinical or symptom factors
4. Contextual or situation variables

Relevant topics for assessment in each of these areas are described in the following sections.

Historical or Developmental Factors

- Family of origin
- Parental instability during childhood
- Parents' parenting style
- Experience of family maltreatment and violence during childhood
- Socialization experiences outside the home
- Exposure to nonfamily violence during childhood
- Exposure to positive supports during childhood
- Social competence
- Educational and academic functioning
- Vocational functioning
- Interpersonal and relational functioning
- Life impulsivity and irresponsibility
- Functioning as a parent
- History of violent behavior
- Intrafamily violence
- History of extrafamilial violence
- Characteristics of prior violence and maltreatment that enhance risk
  — Age at onset
  — Number of prior episodes
  — Duration of pattern
  — Frequency and escalation
  — Number of victims
  — Type of violent behaviors
  — Criminal versatility
  — Threatened or actual use of a weapon

— Threats of injury or death
— Severity and physical injury
— Victim gender
— Precipitating behaviors and motivations
— Consequences and interventions
— Adjustment on conditional release
— Institutional adjustment
• Biological factors

Personal or Dispositional Factors

• Cognitive functioning
• Level of intellectual functioning
• Other cognitive and neurological deficits
— Problem solving
— Abstract reasoning and cognitive flexibility
— Perceptual accuracy
— Attributional styles
— Attitudes and beliefs
• Expectations of child behavior (parent only)
• Emotional functioning
• Sexual functioning
• Personality functioning
— Attachment style
— Apathy
— Domineering, controlling interpersonal style
— Emotional immaturity
— Empathy
— External locus of control
— Impulsivity
— Passive-dependency
— Pervasive anger and hostility
— Self-concept and self-esteem
— Personality disorders
— Psychopathy
• Perceived stress
• Coping responses and internal resources
— Coping skills
— Ability to perceive and access social supports
— Motivation and readiness for change

Clinical or Symptom Factors

- Specific symptoms
- Psychotic illnesses
- Parental psychosis with delusions involving the child
- Command hallucinations or delusions that focus on the child
- Threatening mannerisms, posturing
- Grandiosity
- Suspiciousness
- Agitation
- Character disorders
- Suicidal ideation or behaviors
- More general patterns of violent thoughts or behaviors
- Parental emotional problems and instability
- Dysphoric emotions
- Generalized anger
- Anger and hostility toward women
- Marital anger
- Substance abuse

Current Situation and Contextual Factors

- Victim factors
  — Age
  — Gender
  — Physical, temperamental, and developmental factors
- Social and economic factors
  — Economic poverty
  — Family structure
  — Home environment
  — Residential stability
  — Neighborhood quality
- Child-parent dyad and interactive factors
- Current family functioning and patterns
- Social supports

Conclusions and Recommendations

Melton and colleagues (1997) have strongly cautioned evaluators to recognize that although the professional literature provides some foundation for providing recommendations or, as they described it, "informed speculation about possible dispositional alternatives, the more striking impression about the literature is how much is *not* known" (p. 465). They urge, in response to this, "great humility in making predictions and offering other opinions" (p. 465).

The present authors recommend that the conclusions and recommendations offered in any professional child maltreatment risk assessment evaluation be clinical in nature and not address ultimate legal issues. Although there is controversy about whether evaluators should address ultimate issues when conducting forensic evaluations (American Psychological Association Committee on Professional Practice and Standards, 1998), the recommendation offered here is consistent with others (e.g., Melton et al., 1997) who strongly advise clinicians to avoid addressing ultimate question issues. Inferences about what constitutes the threshold for minimally adequate parenting, what degree of risk to a child warrants out-of-home placement, or what justifies termination of parental rights are not supportable by social scientific data and clinicians have no specific expertise to offer regarding these agency and public policy issues. Such decisions are the responsibility of those empowered to make them and are best left within their province.

Useful clinical findings that fall short of drawing legal conclusions may, however, have a direct bearing on ultimate issue questions. For example, regarding juvenile forensic evaluations, Grisso (1998) noted that clinical findings about an individual's amenability for treatment are directly relevant to ultimate questions before the court, yet they are well within the province of the clinical forensic evaluator. Similarly, descriptions of a child's primary attachments and need for permanency will provide the courts and other decision makers with information that bears directly on the legal questions at hand. This behooves clinicians to be thoughtful and circumspect in the presentation of their data even when they stop short of offering explicit opinions on ultimate legal issues.

Conclusions and recommendations integrating evaluation findings with a clear, clinical analysis of risk factors followed by a set of practical risk management strategies, are most likely to be helpful to those who ultimately are charged with the responsibility to make legal and public policy decisions. In cases involving physically, sexually, and psychologically abusive behaviors, risk factors and risk management interventions pertaining directly to these concerns should be described. Similarly, when chronic physical or psychological neglect is identified, specific ways to address these risk factors should be discussed. It is important that risk assessments identify parental strengths as well as risk factors and vulnerabilities, environmental stresses and supports, and the child's developmental needs and special needs, if present, as well as including a discussion of the parents' abilities to meet these needs.

When children have been referred for assessment of their psychological and behavioral functioning and possible treatment needs, child maltreatment risk assessments should provide recommendations for each referred child in the family according to his or her individual developmental requirements and special needs, if present. Recommendations also should include strategies to reduce symptoms that are related to previous maltreatment as well as interventions that are or may be needed to reduce the risk of negative outcomes which may arise at new developmental stages or may persist.

If a parent presents with deficits that interfere with his or her ability to meet the child's basic developmental needs safely and adequately, the next question concerns prognosis. The question of prognosis, however, is not simply whether the parent can make necessary and appropriate changes to adequately meet his or her child's basic developmental needs, but whether the parent can become able to meet each child's needs within a timeframe that is consistent with the child's developmental requirements.

The Conclusions and Recommendations section of the forensic child maltreatment clinical evaluation report can be divided into two major sections: Risk Assessment and Risk Management.

Risk Assessment

As has been emphasized throughout this guide, child maltreatment and its effects are interactive processes involving both person-specific factors, such as individual competence, and situational variables (Grisso, 1986; Wolfe, 1985). Evaluators must sift through the data to provide a functional assessment of factors associated with the risk of child maltreatment and risk management or, in the case of child assessment, negative sequelae.

Risk factors contributing to the occurrence of maltreatment have been classified as including two broad categories: potentiating factors and compensatory factors (Cicchetti and Rizley, 1981). Potentiating factors are those that increase the likelihood that maltreatment will occur. Compensatory factors are those that decrease the risk of maltreatment.

Risk factors also may be transitory or fluid rather than lasting or unchanging. Various life stresses may be time limited, and there is the possibility, as yet unresearched, that some parents may be better able to meet a child's needs during some developmental periods than others (Milner et al., 1998). As Cicchetti and Toth (1995) noted, "there are *transient* risk factors that fluctuate and may indicate a temporary state. Conversely, there also are enduring factors that represent more permanent conditions or characteristics. According to this transactional model, maltreatment occurs only when potentiating factors outweigh compensatory ones" (p. 544).

Unfortunately, as noted in Chapter 3, the risk for violence is very difficult to predict. Furthermore, as Borum (1996) noted, there currently are no accepted national professional standards or protocols to guide the assessment and management of violence and maltreatment.

In view of the apparent lack of a reliable and valid child maltreatment risk assessment protocol, Grisso's (1998) suggestions regarding juvenile evaluations appear applicable for child maltreatment risk assessments.

> Until actuarial base rates are available . . . risk estimates will have to be based on systematic clinical logic that uses the risk factors described in this . . . [manual]. Reports and testimony about these estimates *must provide a complete description of the data and logic on which they are based* [italics in original]. The court should be given enough information to decide the weight to be given to the evidence and our opinions and should provide attorneys with sufficient information to challenge any of the clinician's assumptions. If the job is done systematically, using multiple sources of data to attend to the full range of risk factors, complete disclosure of the clinician's logic is far more convincing and helpful to the court than an unsupported recitation of one's conclusions. (pp. 156-157)

Core Risk Assessment Questions. Answers to core risk assessment questions provide relevant clinical information needed for effective case management. By providing such information, decision makers, such as judges or child protective workers and supervisors, can exercise their responsibilities to determine what level of risk exists and what official actions are required. The core risk assessment questions include:

- What person-specific and contextual factors may increase risk of maltreatment?
- How frequent or persistent are these factors across time and situations?
- What person-specific and contextual factors mitigate or buffer the risk of maltreatment?
- To what extent can mitigating or buffering factors be facilitated or supported?
- To what extent can risk factors be remedied or managed?

Risk Management Recommendations

Rebalancing the risk assessment equation to enhance child safety and effect positive change may require interventions that reduce risk factors, increase protective factors, or, most likely, do both. Practical and specific treatment recommendations that are directly linked to the identified risk factors for maltreatment are essential.

Parent interventions should focus directly on the factors that increase and decrease the risk of child maltreatment. Interventions should be designed to facilitate the parents' ability to adequately and nonabusively care for and supervise their children. In addition to the specialized interventions described in Chapter 4, consideration should be given to ways of reducing situational demands, creating motivation to effect positive change, increasing life skills and social competence, addressing mental health needs, and directly intervening in maladaptive patterns of behavior. The individual's motivation and ability to utilize and benefit from interventions will require ongoing assessment.

For children, the focus will be upon the factors that are related to the negative effects of child maltreatment and related sequelae as well as other factors that contribute to long-term negative effects and dysfunction which may perpetuate an intergenerational cycle of maltreatment. More specifically:

Interventions with children after abuse experiences must always attend to identifying abuse effects that are compromising important developmental tasks and to promoting normal developmental processes and accomplishments as a primary method of reducing the risk of long-term negative consequences. (Berliner, 1997, p. 161)

Interventions must be individualized because perpetrators and victims of child maltreatment and their individual circumstances vary (Saunders, 1995). Furthermore, individualized interventions are likely to be most effective (Cohn and Daro, 1987) when tailored to the individual's cognitive level and learning style (Andrews et al., 1990). When interventions are not appropriately matched to the needs of the individual or family, this incongruence may lead to erroneous conclusions; for example, that the treatment approach was ineffective, used incorrectly, or that something in the individual or family undermined treatment (Looney, 1984).

Effective intervention is likely to require focusing not only on individual family members but the larger system of family and community relationships as well. For example, interventions may be needed to teach a parent how to nurture and play with his or her children in order to facilitate positive attachments. Reducing social isolation and enhancing social supports and monitoring, for children as well as parents, may also be important components of effective intervention in some cases. Interventions such as in-home support programs, public nursing visits, and school-based services as well as assistance from church and community groups, Big Brothers Big Sisters of America, and similar organizations may also make valuable contributions. In addition to interventions that address child maltreatment risk factors, when specific symptoms such as psychosis, depression, anxiety, and substance abuse are present appropriate mental health treatment may be required to address these difficulties.

To be effective, multilevel interventions may require prioritizing and need to be implemented in ways that do not overwhelm the parent, child, and family (Mosher, 1998; Looney, 1984; Pearce and Pezzot-Pearce, 1997). Once child safety is assured, required initial interventions may include reducing family instability and chaos and providing for the family and its members' basic needs, such as adequate food, shelter, and sleep. In order to reduce the risk of maltreatment, some families may require a comprehensive package of services that provides a range of services for individual family members as well as the family as a whole.

When known, specific services and community resources may be identified within the evaluations to facilitate the appropriate interventions. If possible, multiple options should be provided to avoid possible or perceived conflicts of interest. When appropriate services are not available, this fact should be noted and alternatives to the ideal treatment plan may be offered, while noting their possible benefits and limitations.

One recommendation that is often seen but is generally not very helpful is a generic recommendation for mental health "counseling" or "parenting classes." In fact, "Blindly recommending a short-term parenting group for a chronically troubled, multiproblem family may lead to further failure and frustration for these parents, and it will do little to help their child" (Pearce and Pezzot-Pearce, 1997, p. 71).

CONDUCTING AND WRITING QUALITY EVALUATIONS

Webster and colleagues (1997b) discussed twenty points that contribute to evaluation failure. These items include:

- not clarifying the purpose of the evaluation
- not requiring adequate assessment circumstances
- not establishing and disclosing the limits of one's incompetence
- not acknowledging the possibility of assessor bias
- not utilizing a systematic approach to the evaluation
- not becoming familiar with record files (even when they are voluminous)
- not checking or evaluating the correctness of provided information
- not considering actuarial factors
- not reviewing how the subject or others experienced the event or events in question
- overrelying on psychiatric diagnoses in lieu of current symptomology
- not emphasizing current circumstances
- not considering risk management issues
- not considering base rates

- not providing probabilistic data as to the likelihood of specific types of violence in particular situations and timeframes
- not justifying one's opinions
- not restricting reporting to relevant data
- not obtaining second opinions
- not securing outcome data

Webster and colleagues acknowledged that they advocate a "painstaking" approach, but argued that such a systematic effort is necessary to improve the predictive abilities of risk assessors (p. 354).

Grisso (1998) and others (e.g., Melton et al., 1997) have provided suggestions to facilitate quality forensic report writing. Grisso's recommendations include utilizing a consistent outline and writing clearly and concisely, without clinical jargon. He recommended that all sources of information be listed and that all of the data which form the basis of the evaluator's conclusions and recommendations be included as well. After the data have been described, interpretations and conclusions should follow. Clear explanations for each opinion should be included. Identified problems and recommendations should be presented in a "commonsense manner" so they can be understood by all of the parties involved (Looney, 1984, p. 530). Azar and colleagues (1998) suggested that evaluators might offer the court multiple interpretations of evaluation findings. They noted that a discussion of the strengths and weaknesses of the alternate interpretations may assist judges in making their determinations.

According to the State Forensic Service (1995) of Maine, a quality forensic evaluation

a. Is conducted in an impartial manner and does not advocate for a particular . . . outcome.
b. Communicates concepts clearly and effectively. Explains or avoids clinical jargon.
c. Presents factual basis for concepts and opinions stated in the report.
d. Is timely.
e. Demonstrates sound clinical skills, specialized knowledge . . . Effectively educates non-clinicians about these issues.
f. Evidences satisfactory understanding of forensic issues and the distinction between legal and clinical issues.

g. Is conducted in a manner consistent with the ethics of the clinician's profession. (p. 8)

PROFESSIONAL ISSUES

As previously discussed, child maltreatment evaluations are complex assessments with real-world consequences. A number of professional issues have been discussed throughout this manual. Other issues, such as expert testimony, are beyond the scope of this guide and can be found elsewhere (e.g., Brodsky, 1991, 1999; Grisso, 1998; Melton et al., 1997; Stern, 1997).

This section will address three additional areas that warrant attention. The first area concerns a body of research involving the evaluator's mental processes. These include possible systematic errors in information processing, human judgment, and decision making. The second area involves multicultural issues, which have relevance for intervention as well as assessment. The very important third topic, burnout, concerns the potential negative effects that evaluators may experience as a result of conducting child maltreatment assessments.

Mental Processes

Given the aforementioned limitations of empirical research and clinical practice, child maltreatment evaluations require evaluators to consider these limitations as they combine and synthesize existent scientific knowledge with clinical knowledge to arrive at and present thoughtful and circumspect assessments, judgments, and recommendations to decision makers. Because at the heart of these evaluations is the clinician's role as a gatherer, analyzer, and synthesizer of information, it behooves clinicians to be mindful of their own mental processes.

Mindfulness of one's own mental processes when conducting child maltreatment evaluations is enhanced by an awareness of the work that has been done on identifying systematic errors in information processing, human judgment, and decision making when performing these assessment tasks. More detailed reviews of these issues and their application to forensic and child maltreatment assessments are available elsewhere (e.g., Borum et al., 1993; Poole and Lamb, 1998). A brief summary of the issues follows.

Systematic errors in clinical judgment and decision making are a result of cognitive biases and information processing errors. Such information processing errors and biases include a range of potential problems and difficulties (Borum et al., 1993; Poole and Lamb, 1998). For example, errors frequently occur when practitioners overestimate the strength of the relationship between factors, conditions, or behaviors—sometimes believing a relationship is present when it is not or believing the relationship is in an opposite direction than what actually exists.

Another way information processing difficulties occur depends upon how problems are framed or worded. For example, Poole and Lamb (1998) noted that a finding such as 80 percent of children in a memory study had evidenced accurate recall may be considered a positive finding by some, whereas others may be distressed about how many children were inaccurate in their recall.

Similarly, relationships between factors may be overestimated when conditional probabilities are reversed. As an example of reversing conditional probabilities, Poole and Lamb (1998) used the finding that a substantial proportion of child abusers were abused when they were children. Because many people who were abused do not become abusers, the fact that someone was abused as a child will not, by itself, provide diagnostic or prognostic information. As these authors observed, "Single indicators are rarely diagnostic. Rather, professionals often combine information from multiple indicators that have varying degrees of relationship to the target condition" (p. 216). Such combinations are what risk assessment is all about.

Sometimes evaluators are overconfident about their judgments and may excessively attend to confirmatory information. They also may overrely on initial information and not make necessary adjustments when new, contradictory information is presented (Borum et al., 1993; Poole and Lamb, 1998).

In addition, the personal history characteristics of the evaluator may bias information processing and decision making. For example, research has shown that professionals who were sexually or physically abused as children were more likely to find allegations of sexual abuse believable than were those who had not been abused (Nuttall and Jackson, 1994). Evaluator gender differences also have been observed in some studies, but findings have varied (Milner et al., 1998). Herzberger and Tennen (1985), for example, found that women are more likely to evaluate described disciplinary parent-child situations as inappropriate, severe, abusive, and more likely to result in emotional harm than males did.

The gender of the subject of the evaluation also may affect judgments (Milner et al., 1998). For example, particularly when older victims of child sexual abuse were involved, male perpetrators of child sexual abuse have been considered more responsible for the abuse than female perpetrators (Wagner et al., 1993; Waterman and Foss-Goodman, 1984). In addition, males have attributed increased responsibility to older male victims of child sexual abuse (Waterman and Foss-Goodman, 1984), more responsibility to male victims of child physical abuse than female victims, and also blamed male children more when the abuser was male rather than female (Muller et al., 1993).

Erroneous judgments and decision making also may occur when there is an overreliance on vivid or detailed case-specific information and uncontrolled sources of information, such as clinical experience in the absence of systematic and controlled study (Borum et al., 1993; Poole and Lamb, 1998). Judgment errors also may occur when evaluators overemphasize perceived surface similarities between factors and when evaluators do not consider whether their observations may be the result of chance fluctuations.

A variety of factors contribute to cognitive biases and information processing errors. These problems include overrelying on memory and selective information (Borum et al., 1993; Poole and Lamb, 1998). In addition, opportunities for corrective feedback frequently are limited in applied settings. When feedback occurs it typically is not immediate, systematic, or necessarily free of distortions (Poole and Lamb, 1998).

Various strategies that may enhance clinical judgment and decision making in applied and forensic settings have been suggested (Borum et al., 1993; Poole and Lamb, 1998). For example, Poole and Lamb stated that careful record keeping and familiarity with controlled research is the strongest protection against cognitive biases and information-processing errors. Borum and colleagues suggested that, when writing case notes, evaluators should clearly distinguish between observations and impressions. Poole and Lamb recommended that in addition to maintaining careful records, evaluators should remember that memories are selective and, consequently, refer to their records often.

Evaluation protocols and structured interviews are generally recommended to facilitate assessment procedures (Borum, 1996; Milner et al., 1998). These evaluation strategies can remind evaluators to probe areas they may otherwise have neglected and by doing so, may provide more reliable information and enhance predictive accuracy. Yet, the validity of such interview approaches will depend on a number of factors. These factors include whether the interviewer has had training in general interviewing skills and in interviewing people about difficult and sensitive issues, as well as whether the interviewer adheres to the interview protocol (Milner et al., 1998). Additional risks to the validity of any interview approach include the information-processing errors described above.

Additional approaches for reducing information-processing and clinical judgment errors include testing multiple and alternative hypotheses, searching for disconfirming information, considering the flip side of problems, and being sure to consider the less vivid, more common information (Borum et al., 1993; Poole and Lamb, 1998). Evaluators also are encouraged to write down their hypotheses and list alternative hypotheses and information that call the evaluator's preferred hypotheses into question.

In order to reduce cognitive biases and information-processing errors, evaluators need to keep current with the empirical literature and, when possible, determine the strength of the relationships between factors to ascertain how well relevant variables discriminate between categories or groups. Poole and Lamb (1998) also suggested that professionals who conduct such work should periodically reevaluate their beliefs and opinions and think about new information and previously available information as a whole.

When engaging in predictive judgments, base rate information detailing the prevalence of characteristics or behaviors in a population is very important for reducing cognitive errors and biases. As Borum and colleagues (1993) recommend:

> . . . the first step is to identify the population to which the predictee belongs and then attempt to identify the base rates of the behavior of interest within that population. Whenever possible, the forensic clinician should use those norms that are most appropriate for the individual case. . . . Absent such specific

base rate information, the clinician should consider base rates of similar behaviors or base rates of the behavior of interest in other, similar populations . . . the examiner can then consider assessment data and (cautiously) modify these rates accordingly to make a judgment about the individual case. (pp. 45-46)

It is important to remember that child abuse risk assessments occur within a stressful and often emotional context. The pressures to assure child safety yet preserve family attachments are great. Evaluators "can help ensure that their work meets ethical, professional, and scientific standards by regularly consulting with respected colleagues" while maintaining legal and professional standards of confidentiality (Saunders, 1997, p. 137).

Multicultural Issues

Special difficulties may arise in child maltreatment evaluations when the family or child being assessed belongs to an ethnic, cultural, or racial minority group. In practice, it is the burden of the evaluator to determine if and when ethnic or cultural factors are likely to impinge on the effectiveness and fairness of a child maltreatment evaluation. Early in the assessment, the evaluator must determine the extent to which the client has assimilated the dominant culture or is functioning within a traditional cultural framework (Dana, 2000). The evaluator must learn about the client's cultural practices, including such matters as family structure patterns, child-rearing practices, and gender-role issues (Abney, 2002; American Psychological Association [APA], 1993). The evaluator must determine whether a language barrier exists that has the potential for affecting the outcome of the evaluation (Preciado and Henry, 1997), and he or she must secure appropriate, professional interpretation services when necessary in order to ensure comprehension in the evaluation process (APA, 1993). The evaluator must be sensitive to cultural dimensions of the abuse allegations themselves and be aware of current child welfare and criminal legal standards regarding the use of cultural evidence in the courtroom as mitigating factors (Levesque, 2000).

The evaluator also must determine whether the assessment methods typically used are appropriate for the individual or family in question and whether studies exist supporting the valid use of the measures with individuals from that particular ethnic, cultural, or national background (Dana, 2000). To make such a determination, the evaluator will need to consult a growing body of empirical research literature concerning the crosscultural uses of standard psychometric instruments (e.g., Dana, 1998; Hall et al., 1999; Kwan, 1999; Negy and Snyder, 2000; Okazaki and Sue, 2000). The ethical standards of the American Psychological Association (1992) require that psychologists be aware of the limitations of the assessment instruments they use to reach diagnoses and predictions about individuals. Ethical standard 2.04(c) requires in particular that psychologists be alert to situations in which assessment methods or the norms they are based on may not be applicable or may need adjustment because of such factors as race, ethnicity, national origin, language, and so on. The American Psychological Association's "Guidelines for Providers of Psychological Services to Individuals from Culturally Diverse Populations" (1993) also details a wide range of multicultural concerns, including language barriers, that the provider must address. Similarly, the Standards for Educational and Psychological Testing (AERA, APA, and NCME, 1999) require that psychometric tests be used in a culturally and linguistically fair manner.

Given the fact that child maltreatment evaluations often inform decisions that have a profound impact on children and their families, in a multicultural context the evaluator is advised to take a conservative position and to highlight only those findings which are clearly supported by the data, given the many levels of cultural and ethnic variables that may be operating in the background to the evaluation process. As a simple example, many immigrant and refugee populations come from cultures where the threat of social stigma makes it extremely difficult to acknowledge *any* emotional problems such as depression or anxiety. The evaluator must be careful not to classify such reticence as evidence of a higher-than-usual level of defensiveness about personal problems, for such a conclusion based on a cultural variable alone might adversely affect a decision or outcome. Careful vigilance and sensitivity to cultural factors is required in child maltreatment evaluations.

Fighting Burnout

Conducting child maltreatment evaluations can be very taxing. Studies have demonstrated that professionals who work with people who have experienced or perpetrated child maltreatment and sexual violence may suffer deleterious effects that may negatively impact their work (Lyons, 1993; Thorpe et al., 2001). For example, Lyons found that some hospital staff working with people who have child maltreatment histories experienced severe negative reactions to their patients' accounts of their experiences of abuse and violence; such reactions included nightmares, repetitive and intrusive images, and somatic problems. Staff support was considered instrumental in helping these staff members to effectively manage their reactions, maintain effective boundaries, and do their work. Some staff found that as they became more able to maintain their personal boundaries they experienced greater empathy, increased creativity, enhanced spiritual or moral awareness, and more energy to continue to do this important work.

Various coping strategies may help professionals manage the negative effects that can occur when working in the area of child abuse and neglect (Figley, 1995; Pearce and Pezzot-Pearce, 1997; Thorpe et al., 2001). In addition to establishing supportive collegial relationships, strategies include being aware of personal issues and attitudes that can negatively affect one's work, obtaining appropriate training and continuing educational experiences, limiting the number of cases involving child maltreatment, and maintaining a safe working environment and practice. More broadly, maintaining active, healthy personal lives that are separate from one's work and having a sense of humor despite repeated exposure to the face of human adversity are essential. By managing the negative impact of this work, people working in this important area can experience the professional and personal rewards that accompany these endeavors.

References

Abel, G. G., Becker, J. V., Murphy, W. D., and Flanagan, B. (1981). Identifying dangerous child molesters. In R. Stuart (Ed.), *Violent behavior: Social learning approaches to prediction, management and treatment* (pp. 116-137). New York: Brunner-Mazel.

Abel, G. G., Mittleman, M., Becker, J. V., Rathner, J., and Rouleau, J. L. (1988). Predicting child molesters' response to treatment. In R. A. Prenky and V. L. Quinsey (Eds.). *Human sexual aggression: Current perspectives* (pp. 223-234). New York: The New York Academy of Sciences.

Abernathy, S., Alexander, D., and Brooks, J. (1998). Do risk instruments matter? Is having completed a risk assessment instrument correlated with having addressed risk issues in the casework, A Tennessee example. In J. Fluke, R. Alsop, and C. Race (Eds.), *Twelfth national roundtable on child protective services risk assessment: Summary of proceedings* (pp. 1-2). Englewood, CO: American Humane Association.

Abidin, R. R. (1995). *Parenting stress index,* Third edition. *Odessa, FL: Psychological Assessment Resources.*

Abney, V.D. (2002). Cultural competency in the field of child maltreatment. In J. Myers, L. Berliner, J. Briere, J. C. T. Hendrix, C. Jenny, and T. Reid (Eds.). *The APSAC handbook on child maltreatment,* Second edition (pp. 477-487). Thousand Oaks, CA: Sage Publications.

Achenbach, T. M. (1991). *Manual for the child behavior checklist/4-18 and 1991 profile.* Burlington, VT: University of Vermont, Department of Psychiatry.

Ackerman, M. J. (1999). *Essentials of forensic psychological assessment.* New York: John Wiley and Sons, Inc.

Adoption and Safe Families Act, Pub. L. No. 105-89, 111 Stat. 2115, (1997).

Ageton, S. S. (1983). *Sexual assault among adolescents.* Lexington, MA: Lexington Books.

Aldarondo, E. and Sugarman, D. B. (1996). Risk marker analysis of the cessation and persistence of wife assault. *Journal of Consulting and Clinical Psychology, 64*(5), 1010-1019.

Alksnis, C. and Taylor, J. (1994). The impact of experiencing and witnessing family violence during childhood: Child and adult behavioural outcomes (online). Correctional Service Canada: www.csc-scc.gc.ca/text/pblct/fv/fv04/toce.shtml.

Altemeier, W. A. III, O'Conner, S., Vietze, P. M., Sandler, H. M., and Sherrod, K. B. (1982). Antecedents of child abuse. *Behavioral Pediatrics, 100*(5), 823-829.

American Academy of Child and Adolescent Psychiatry (1997). Practice parameters for the forensic evaluation of children and adolescents who may have been physically or sexually abused. *Journal of the American Academy of Child and Adolescent Psychiatry, 36*(10), (Suppl.), 37S-56S.

American Academy of Psychiatry and the Law (1995). Ethical Guidelines for the Practice of Forensic Psychiatry (online). www. aapl.org/ethics.htm.

American Bar Association (1998). *ASFA overview*. Washington, DC: American Bar Association.

American Educational Research Association, American Psychological Association, and National Council on Measurement in Education (1999). *The standards for educational and psychological testing*. Washington, DC: AERA Publications Sales.

American Professional Society on the Abuse of Children (1995a). *Practice guidelines: Use of anatomical dolls in child sexual abuse assessments*. Chicago: Author.

American Professional Society on the Abuse of Children (1995b). *Psychosocial evaluation of suspected psychological maltreatment in children and adolescents*. Chicago: Author.

American Professional Society on the Abuse of Children (1997). *Guidelines for psychosocial evaluations of suspected sexual abuse in young children*. Chicago: Author.

American Psychological Association (1992). Ethical principles of psychologists and code of conduct. *American Psychologist, 47*(12), 1597-1611.

American Psychological Association (1993). Guidelines for providers of psychological services to ethnic, linguistic, and culturally diverse populations. *American Psychologist, 48*(1), 45-48.

American Psychological Association Committee on Professional Practice and Standards (1998). *Guidelines for psychological evaluations in child protection matters*. Washington, DC: American Psychological Association.

Ammerman, R. T. (1998). Methodological issues in child maltreatment research. In J. R. Lutzker (Ed.), *Handbook of child abuse research and treatment: Issues in clinical child psychology* (pp. 117-132). New York: Plenum Press.

Ammerman, R. T., Herson, M., Van Hasselt, V. B., Lubetsky, M. J., and Sieck, W. R. (1994). Maltreatment in psychiatrically hospitalized children and adolescents with developmental disabilities: Prevalence and correlates. *Journal of the American Academy of Child and Adolescent Psychiatry, 33*(4), 567-576.

Andrews, D. A., Bonta, J., and Hoge, R. D. (1990). Classification for effective rehabilitation: Rediscovering psychology. *Criminal Justice and Behavior, 17*(1), 19-52.

Araji, S. (1997). *Sexually aggressive children: Coming to understand them*. Thousand Oaks, CA: Sage Publications.

Araji, S. and Finkelhor, D. (1985). Explanations of pedophilia: Review of empirical research. *The Bulletin of the American Academy of Psychiatry and the Law, 13*(1), 17-37.

Association for the Treatment of Sexual Abusers (2001). *Practice standards and guidelines for members of the Association for the Treatment of Sexual Abusers.* Beaverton, OR: Author.

Azar, S. T. (1989). Training parents of abused children. In C. E. Schaefer and J. M. Briesmeister (Eds.), *Handbook of parent training* (pp. 414-441). New York: Wiley.

Azar, S. T. (1996, June). "Termination of parental rights evaluation in child abuse and neglect cases: Can behavioral science help Solomon?" Presentation sponsored by the Continuing Health Education Partnership, Inc., Augusta, ME.

Azar, S. T. (1997). A cognitive behavioral approach to understanding and treating parents who physically abuse their children. In D. A. Wolfe, R. J. McMahon, and R. DeV. Peters (Eds.), *Child abuse: New directions in prevention and treatment across the lifespan* (pp. 79-101). Thousand Oaks, CA: Sage Publications.

Azar, S. T., Benjet, C. L., Fuhrmann, G. S., and Cavallero, L. (1995). Child maltreatment and termination of parental rights: Can behavioral research help Solomon? *Behavior Therapy, 26*(4), 599-623.

Azar, S. T., Lauretti, A. F., and Loding, B. V. (1998). The evaluation of parental fitness in termination of parental rights cases: A functional-contextual perspective. *Clinical Child and Family Psychology Review, 1*(2), 77-100.

Azar, S. T., Robinson, D. R., Hekimian, E., and Twentyman, C. T. (1984). Unrealistic expectations and problem-solving ability in maltreating and comparison mothers. *Journal of Consulting and Clinical Psychology, 52*(4), 687-691.

Azar, S. T. and Wolfe, D. A. (1998). Child physical abuse and neglect. In E. J. Mash, and R. A. Barkley (Eds.), *Treatment of childhood disorders,* Second edition (pp. 501-544). New York: The Guilford Press.

Banyard, V. (1999). Childhood maltreatment and the mental health of low-income women. *American Journal of Orthopsychiatry, 69*(2), 161-171.

Barbaree, H. E. and Marshall, W. L. (1988). Deviant sexual arousal, offense history, and demographic variables as predictors of reoffense among child molesters. *Behavioral Sciences and the Law, 6*(2), 267-280.

Barbaree, H. E., Seto, M. C., Serin, R. C., Amos, H. L., and Preston, D. L. (1994). Comparisons between sexual and nonsexual rapist subtypes: Sexual arousal to rape, offense precursors, and offense characteristics. *Criminal Justice and Behavior, 21*(1) 95-114.

Barnett, D., Manly, J. T., and Cicchetti, D. (1994). Defining child maltreatment: The interface between policy and research. In D. Cicchetti and S. L. Toth (Eds.), *Child abuse, child development, and social policy: Advances in applied developmental psychology,* Vol. 8 (pp. 7-73). Norwood, NJ: Ablex Publishing Corporation.

Barnum, R. (1997). A suggested framework for forensic consultation in cases of child abuse and neglect. *Journal of the American Academy of Psychiatry and the Law, 25*(4), 581-593.

Bates, J. E. and Bayles, K. (1988). Attachment and the development of behavior problems. In J. Belsky and T. Nezworski (Eds.), *Clinical Implications of Attachment* (pp. 253-299). Hillsdale, NJ: Lawrence Erlbaum Associates.

Bath, H. I. and Haapala, D. A. (1993). Intensive family preservation services with abused and neglected children: An examination of group differences. *Child Abuse and Neglect, 17*(2), 213-225.

Baumeister, R. F., Smart, L., and Boden, J. M. (1996). Relation of threatened egotism to violence and aggression: The dark side of high self-esteem. *Psychological Review, 103*(1), 5-33.

Becker, J. V. (1998). What we know about the characteristics and treatment of adolescents who have committed sexual offenses. *Child Maltreatment, 3*(4), 317-329.

Becker, J. V., Alpert, J. L., BigFoot, D. S., Bonner, B. L., Geddie, L. F., Henggeler, S. W., Kaufman, K. L., and Walker, C. E. (1995). Empirical research on child abuse treatment: Report by the Child Abuse and Neglect Treatment Working Group, American Psychological Association. *Journal of Clinical Child Psychology, 24*(Suppl.), 23-46.

Becker, J. V. and Hunter, J. A. Jr. (1997). Understanding and treating child and adolescent sexual offenders. In T. H. Ollendick and R. J. Prinz (Eds.), *Advances in Clinical Child Psychology,* Vol. 19, (pp. 177-197). New York: Plenum Press.

Becker, J. V. and Murphy, W. D. (1998). What we know and do not know about assessing and treating sex offenders. *Psychology, Public Policy, and Law, 4*(1-2), 116-138.

Bell, P. and Wagner, D. (1998). The use of the risk assessment to evaluate the impact of intensive protective service intervention in a practice setting. In J. Fluke, R. Alsop, and C. Race (Eds.), *Twelfth national roundtable on child protective services risk assessment: Summary of proceedings* (pp. 3-10). Englewood, CO: American Humane Association.

Belsky, J. (1980). Child maltreatment: An ecological integration. *American Psychologist, 35*(4), 320-335.

Belsky, J. (1993). Etiology of child maltreatment: A developmental-ecological analysis. *Psychological Bulletin, 114*(3), 413-434.

Bennett, S. E., Hughes, H. M., and Luke, D. A. (2000). Heterogeneity in patterns of child sexual abuse, family functioning, and long-term adjustment. *Journal of Interpersonal Violence, 15*(2), 134-157.

Berenbaum, H. (1999). Peculiarity and reported child maltreatment. *Psychiatry, 62*(1), 21-35.

Berliner, L. (1996). Intervening in domestic violence: Should victims and offenders or couples be the focus? *Journal of Interpersonal Violence, 11*(3), 449-450.

Berliner, L. (1997). Trauma-specific therapy for sexually abused children. In D. A. Wolfe, R. J. McMahon, and R. DeV. Peters (Eds.), *Child abuse: New directions in prevention and treatment across the lifespan* (pp. 157-176). Thousand Oaks, CA: Sage Publications.

Berliner, L. and Elliott, D. M. (2002). Sexual abuse of children. In J. Briere, L. Berliner, J. A. Bulkley, C. Jenny, and T. Reid (Eds.), *The APSAC handbook on child maltreatment*, Second edition (pp. 51-71). Thousand Oaks, CA: Sage Publications.

Berliner, L. and Saunders, B. E. (1996). Treating fear and anxiety in sexually abused children: Results of a controlled 2-year follow-up study. *Child Maltreatment, 1*(4), 294-309.

Berliner, L., Schram, D., Miller, L. L., and Milloy, C. D. (1995). A sentencing alternative for sex offenders: A study of decision making and recidivism. *Journal of Interpersonal Violence, 10*(4), 487-502.

Bishop, S. J. and Leadbeater, B. J. (1999). Maternal social support patterns and child maltreatment: Comparison of maltreating and nonmaltreating mothers. *American Orthopsychiatry, 69*(2), 172-181.

Blumenthal, S., Gudjonsson, G., and Burns, J. (1999). Cognitive distortions and blame attributions in sex offenders against adults and children. *Child Abuse and Neglect, 23*(2), 129-143.

Boer, D. P., Hart, S. D., Kropp, P. R., and Webster, C. D. (1997). *Manual for the sexual violence risk-20*. Vancouver, British Columbia, Canada: The British Columbia Institute Against Family Violence.

Borum, R. (1996). Improving the clinical practice of violence risk assessment: Technology, guidelines, and training. *American Psychologist, 51*(9), 945-956.

Borum, R., Otto, R, and Golding, S. (1993, Spring). Improving clinical judgment and decision making in forensic evaluation. *The Journal of Psychiatry and Law, 21*(1), 35-76.

Bourke, M. L. and Donohue, B. (1996). Assessment and treatment of juvenile sex offenders: An empirical review. *Journal of Child Sexual Abuse, 5*(1), 47-70.

Bower, G. H. (1981). Mood and memory. *American Psychologist, 36*(2), 129-148.

Bowker, L. H., Arbitell, M., and McFerron, J. R. (1988). On the relationship between wife beating and child abuse. In K. Yllö and M. Bograd (Eds.), *Feminist perspectives on wife abuse* (pp. 158-174). Newbury Park, CA: Sage Publications, Inc.

Bradley, E. J. and Peters, R. D. (1991). Physically abusive and nonabusive mothers' perceptions of parenting and child behavior. *American Journal of Orthopsychiatry, 61*(3), 455-460.

Briere, J. (1996). *Trauma symptom checklist for children: Professional manual (TSCC)*. Lutz, FL: Psychological Assessment Resources, Inc.

Briere, J. N. and Elliott, D. M. (1994). Immediate and long-term impacts of child sexual abuse: *The Future of Children. Sexual Abuse of Children, 4*(2), 54-69.

Brodsky, S. (1991). *Testifying in court: Guidelines and maxims for the expert witness*. Washington, DC: American Psychological Association.

Brodsky, S. (1999). *The expert expert witness: More maxims and guidelines for testifying in court*. Washington, DC: American Psychological Association.

Brown, A. and Finkelhor, D. (1986). Initial and long-term effects: A review of the research. In D. Finkelhor, S. Araji, L. Baron, A. Brown, S. D. Peters, and G. E. Wyatt (Eds.), *A sourcebook on child sexual abuse* (pp. 143-179). Beverly Hills: Sage Publications.

Brown, J., Cohen, P., Johnson, J. G., and Salzinger, S. (1998). A longitudinal analysis of risk factors for child maltreatment: Findings of a 17-year prospective study of officially recorded and self-reported child abuse and neglect. *Child Abuse and Neglect, 22*(11), 1065-1078.

Budd, K. S. and Holdsworth, M. J. (1996). Issues in clinical assessment of minimal parenting competence. *Journal of Clinical Child Psychology, 25*(1), 2-14.

Budd, K. S., Poindexter, L. M., and Felix, E. D. (2001). Clinical assessment of parents in child protection cases: An empirical analysis. *Law and Human Behavior, 25*(1), 93-108.

Burton, D. L. (2000). Were adolescent sexual offenders children with sexual behavior problems? *Sexual Abuse: A Journal of Research and Treatment, 12*(1), 37-48.

Butler, S. M., Radia, N., and Magnatta, M. (1994). Maternal compliance to court-ordered assessment in cases of child maltreatment. *Child Abuse and Neglect, 18*(2), 203-211.

Campbell, J. C. (1995). Prediction of homicide of and by battered women. In J. C. Campbell (Ed.), *Assessing dangerousness: Violence by sexual offenders, batterers, and child abusers* (pp. 96-113). Thousand Oaks, CA: Sage Publications.

Campbell, J. C. and Alford, P. (1989). The dark consequences of marital rape. *American Journal of Nursing, 7,* 946-949.

Caplan, P. J., Watters, J., White, G., Parry, R., and Bates, R. (1984). Toronto multiagency child abuse research project: The abused and the abuser. *Child Abuse and Neglect, 8*(3), 343-351.

Carlson, E. A. (1998). A prospective longitudinal study of attachment disorganization/disorientation. *Child Development, 69*(4), 1107-1128.

Carlson, V., Cicchetti, D., Barnett, D., and Braunwald, K. G. (1989). Finding order in disorganization: Lessons from research on maltreated infants' attachments to their caregivers. In D. Cicchetti and V. Carlson (Eds.), *Child maltreatment: Theory and research on the causes and consequences of child abuse and neglect* (pp. 494-528). London: Cambridge University Press.

Catwell, H. B. (1997). The neglect of child neglect. In M. E. Helfer, R. S. Kempe, and R. D. Krugman (Eds.), *The battered child,* Fifth edition (pp. 347-373). Chicago: The University of Chicago Press.

Ceci, S. J. and Hembrooke, H. (1998). *Expert witnesses in child abuse cases: What can and should be said in court.* Washington, DC: American Psychological Association.

Chaffin, M. (1994). Research in action: Assessment and treatment of child sexual abusers. *Journal of Interpersonal Violence, 9*(2), 224-237.

Chaffin, M. and Bonner, B. (1998). Don't shoot, we're your children: Have we gone too far in our response to adolescent sexual abusers and children with sexual behavior problems? *Child Maltreatment, 3*(4), 314-316.

Chamberlain, P. and Moore, K. (1998). A clinical model for parenting juvenile offenders: A comparison of group care versus family care. *Clinical Child Psychology and Psychiatry, 3*(3), 375-386.

Chamberlain, P. and Reid, J. B. (1998). Comparison of two community alternatives to incarceration for chronic juvenile offenders. *Journal of Consulting and Clinical Psychology, 66*(4), 624-633.

Chilamkurti, C. and Milner, J. S. (1993). Perceptions and evaluations of child transgressions and disciplinary techniques in high- and low-risk mothers and their children. *Child Development, 64*, 1801-1814.

Child and Family Services and Child Protection Act (1998). Title 22. Maine Revised Statutes Annotated, Chapter 1071.

Child Assessment News (1998). The assessment of parent-child interactions: Research and controversy, *Child Assessment News, 6*(6), 1, 4, 5, 8, 9.

Child Assessment News (1999). Current concerns in the clinical assessment of child sexual abuse. *Child Assessment News, 7*(2), 1, 4, 5, 8-11.

Christensen, M. J., Brayden, R. M., Dietrich, M. S., McLaughlin, F. J., Sherrod, K. B., and Altemeier, W. A. (1994). The prospective assessment of self-concept in neglectful and physically abusive low-income mothers. *Child Abuse and Neglect, 18*(3), 225-232.

Cicchetti, D. and Lynch, M. (1993). Toward an ecological/transactional model of community violence and child maltreatment: Consequences for children's development. *Psychiatry, 56*(1), 96-118.

Cicchetti, D. and Rizley, R. (1981). Developmental perspectives on the etiology, intergenerational transmission, and sequelae of child maltreatment. *New Directions for Child Development, 11*, 31-55.

Cicchetti, D. and Toth, S. L. (1995). A developmental psychopathology perspective on child abuse and neglect. *Journal of American Academy of Child and Adolescent Psychiatry, 34*(5), 541-565.

Cicchetti, D., Toth, S. L., and Lynch, M. (1995). Bowlby's dream comes full circle: The application of attachment theory to risk and psychopathology. *Advances in Clinical Child Psychology, 17*, 1-74.

Clark, R. (1985). "The Parent-Child Early Relational Assessment." University of Wisconsin Medical School at Madison.

Claussen, A. H. and Crittenden, P. M. (1991). Physical and psychological maltreatment: Relations among types of maltreatment. *Child Abuse and Neglect, 15*(1-2), 5-18.

Coffey, P., Leitenberg, H., Henning, K., Turner, T., and Bennett, R. T. (1996). Mediators of the long-term impact of child sexual abuse: Perceived stigma, betrayal, powerlessness, and self-blame. *Child Abuse and Neglect, 20*(5), 447-455.

Cohen, J. A. and Mannarino, A. P. (1997). A treatment study for sexually abused preschool children: Outcome during a one-year follow-up. *Journal of the American Academy of Child and Adolescent Psychiatry, 36*(9), 1228-1235.

Cohen, J. A. and Mannarino, A. P. (1998). Interventions for sexually abused children: Initial treatment outcome findings. *Child Maltreatment, 3*(1), 17-26.

Cohn, A. H. (1979). Essential elements of successful child abuse and neglect treatment. *Child Abuse and Neglect, 3*(2), 491-496.

Cohn, A. H. and Daro, D. D. (1987). Is treatment too late: What ten years of evaluative research tell us. *Child Abuse and Neglect, 11*(3), 433-442.

Committee on Ethical Guidelines for Forensic Psychologists (1991). Specialty guidelines for forensic psychologists. *Law and Human Behavior, 15*(6), 655-665.

Comstock, G. (1992). Television and film violence. In M. Biskup and C. P. Cozic (Eds.), *Youth Violence* (178-218). San Diego, CA: Greenhaven Press.

Crittenden, P. M. (1985a). Maltreated infants: Vulnerability and resilience. *Journal of Child Psychology and Psychiatry, 26*(1), 85-96.

Crittenden, P. M. (1985b). Social networks, quality of child rearing, and child development. *Child Development, 56*, 1299-1313.

Crittenden, P. M. (1988). Relationships at risk. In J. Belsky and T. Nezworski (Eds.), *Clinical Implications of Attachment* (pp. 136-174). Hillsdale, NJ: Lawrence Erlbaum Associates.

Crittenden, P. M. (1993). An information-processing perspective on the behavior of neglectful parents. *Criminal Justice and Behavior, 20*(1), 27-48.

Crittenden, P. M. (1996). Research on maltreating families: Implications for intervention. In J. Briere, L. Berliner, J. A. Bulkley, C. Jenny, and T. Reid (Eds.), *The APSAC handbook on child maltreatment* (pp. 158-174). Thousand Oaks, CA: Sage Publications.

Crittenden, P. M. (1999). Child neglect: Causes and contributors. In H. Dubowitz (Ed.), *Neglected children: Research, practice, and policy* (pp. 47-68). Thousand Oaks, CA: Sage Publications.

Crouch, J. L. and Milner, J. (1993). Effects of child neglect on children. *Criminal Justice and Behavior, 20*(1), 49-65.

Culbertonson, J. L. and Willis, D. J. (1998). Interventions with young children who have been multiply abused. *Journal of Aggression, Maltreatment and Trauma, 2*(1), 207-232.

Cullen, M. and Freeman-Longo, R. E. (1996). *Men and anger: Understanding and managing your anger for a much better life.* Brandon, VT: The Safer Society Press.

Culp, R. E., Heide, J., and Richardson, M. T. (1987). Maltreated children's developmental scores: Treatment versus nontreatment. *Child Abuse and Neglect, 11*(1), 29-34.

Culp, R. E., Little, V., Letts, D., and Lawrence, H. (1991). Maltreated children's self-concept: Effects of a comprehensive treatment program. *American Journal of Orthopsychiatry, 61*(1), 114-121.

Curran, T. F. (1996). Legal issues in the use of CPS risk assessment instruments. *The APSAC Advisor, 8*(4), 15-20.

Cutrona, C. E. (1984). Social support and stress in the transition to parenthood. *Journal of Abnormal Psychology, 93*(4), 378-390.

Dana, R. H. (1998). Projective assessment of Latinos in the United States: Current realities, problems, and prospects. *Cultural Diversity and Mental Health, 4*(3), 165-184.

Dana, R. H. (2000). Psychological assessment in the diagnosis and treatment of ethnic group members. In J.F. Aponte and J. Wohl (Eds.), *Psychological intervention and cultural diversity* (pp. 59-74). Boston: Allyn and Bacon.

Danoff, N. L., Kemper, K. J., and Sherry, B. (1994). Risk factors for dropping out of a parenting education program. *Child Abuse and Neglect, 18,* 599-606.

Daro, D. (1988). *Confronting child abuse: Research for effective program design.* New York: The Free Press.

Daro, D. (1996). The use of risk assessment in child abuse prevention. *The APSAC Advisor, 8*(4), 11-14.

Daro, D. and McCurdy, K. (1994). Preventing child abuse and neglect: Programmatic interventions. *Child Welfare, LXXIII*(5), 405-430.

Daubert v. Merrell-Dow Pharmaceuticals, Inc., 509 U.S. 579 (1993).

de Paúl, J. and Arruabarrena, M. I. (1995). Behavior problems in school-aged physically abused and neglected children in Spain. *Child Abuse and Neglect, 19*(4), 409-418.

Deblinger, E., Lippmann, J., and Steer, R. (1996). Sexually abused children suffering post-traumatic stress symptoms: Initial treatment outcome findings. *Child Maltreatment, 1*(4), 310-321.

Deblinger, E., Steer, R., and Lippmann, J. (1999). Maternal factors associated with sexually abused children's psychosocial adjustment. *Child Maltreatment, 4*(1), 13-20.

Della Femina, D., Yeager, C. A., and Lewis, D. O. (1990). Child abuse: Adolescent records vs. adult recall. *Child Abuse and Neglect, 14*(2), 227-231.

DePanfilis, D. (1996a). Social isolation of neglectful families: A review of social support assessment and intervention models. *Child Maltreatment, 1*(1), 37-52.

DePanfilis, D. (1996b). Implementing child mistreatment risk assessment systems: Lessons from theory. *Administration in Social Work, 20*(2), 41-59.

DePanfilis, D. (1999). Intervening with families when children are neglected. In H. Dubowitz (Ed.), *Neglected children: Research, practice, and policy* (pp. 211-236). Thousand Oaks, CA: Sage Publications.

DePanfilis, D., and Zuravin, S. J. (1998). Rates, patterns, and frequency of child maltreatment recurrences among families known to CPS. *Child Maltreatment, 3*(1), 27-42.

Dewhurst, A. M. and Nielsen, K. (1997). "Relapse prevention and the transtheoretical model of change: A multidisciplinary, community-based approach to working with conditionally released sexual offenders." Symposium conducted at the Association for the Treatment of Sexual Abusers' 16th Annual 1997 Research and Treatment Conference, Arlington, VA, October.

Diaz, R. M., Neal, C. J., and Vachio, A. (1991). Maternal teaching in the zone of proximal development: A comparison of low- and high-risk dyads. *Merrill-Palmer Quarterly, 37*(1), 83-107.

DiLillo, D. and Long, P. J. (1999). Perceptions of couple functioning among female survivors of child sexual abuse. *Journal of Child Sexual Abuse, 7*(4), 59-76.

Dishion, T. J., McCord, J., Pouli, F. (1999). When interventions harm. Peer groups and problem behavior. *American Psychologist, 54*(9), 755-764.

Doueck, H. J. and Lyons, P. (1998). The Child Well-Being Scales as a predictor of caseworker attention and services in child protection: A preliminary analysis. In J. Fluke, R. Alsop, and C. Race (Eds.), *Twelfth national roundtable on child protective services risk assessment: Summary of proceedings* (pp. 131-144). Englewood, CO: American Humane Association.

Dougher, M. J. (1995). Clinical assessment of sex offenders. In B. Schwartz and H. R. Cellini (Eds.). *The sex offender: Corrections, treatment and legal practice* (pp. 11-1 – 11-13). Kingston, NJ: Civic Research Institute, Inc.

Drach, K. M., Wientzen, J. and Ricci, L. R. (2001). The diagnostic utility of sexual behavior problems in diagnosing sexual abuse in a forensic child abuse evaluation clinic. *Child Abuse and Neglect, 25*(4), 489-503.

Ducharme, J., Koverola, C., and Battle, P. (1997). Intimacy development: the influence of abuse and gender. *Journal of Interpersonal Violence, 12*(4), 590-599.

Dumas, J. E. and Albin, J. B. (1986). Parent training outcome: Does active parental involvement matter? *Behaviour Research and Therapy, 24*(2), 227-230.

Dutton, D. G. (1995). Intimate abusiveness. *Clinical Psychology: Science and Practice, 2*(3), 207-224.

Dutton, D. G. (1996, August). "Batterers and the domestic assault of women." Symposium conducted at Violence and Criminality: A Gathering of Leading Experts. San Diego, CA.

Dutton, D. G. and Hart, S. D. (1992a). Evidence for long-term, specific effects of childhood abuse and neglect on criminal behavior in men. *International Journal of Offender Therapy and Comparative Criminology, 36*(2), 130-137.

Dutton, D. G. and Hart, S. D. (1992b). Risk markers for family violence in a federally incarcerated population. *International Journal of Law and Psychiatry, 15*(1), 101-112.

Dutton, D. G., van Ginkel, C., and Starzomski, A. (1995). The role of shame and guilt in the intergenerational transmission of abusiveness. *Violence and Victims, 10*(2), 121-131.

Dyer, F. J. (1999). *Psychological consultation in parental rights cases.* New York: The Guilford Press.

Edleson, J. L. (1999a). Children's witnessing of adult domestic violence. *Journal of Interpersonal Violence, 14*(8), 839-870.

Edleson, J. L. (Ed.) (1999b). Interventions and issues in the co-occurrence of child abuse and domestic violence. [Special focus issue]. *Child Maltreatment, 4*(2).

Edleson, J. L. and Syers, M. (1991). The effects of group treatment for men who batter: An 18-month follow-up study. *Research on Social Work Practice, 1*(3), 227-243.

Egeland, B. (1988). Breaking the cycle of abuse: Implications for prediction and intervention. In K. D. Browne, C. Davies, and P. Stratton (Eds.), *Early prediction and prevention of child abuse* (pp. 87-99). Chichester, England, UK: John Wiley and Sons Ltd.

Egeland, B. (1993). A history of abuse is a major risk factor for abusing the next generation. In R. Gelles and D. Loseke (Eds.), *Current controversies on family violence* (pp. 197-208). Newbury Park, CA: Sage Publications.

Egeland, B. (1997). Mediators of the effects of child maltreatment on developmental adaptation in adolescence. In D. Cicchetti and S. L. Toth (Eds.), *Rochester Symposium on Developmental Psychopathology.* Vol. VIII, *Developmental perspectives on trauma: Theory, research, and intervention* (pp. 403-434). Rochester, NY: University of Rochester Press.

Egeland, B., Erickson, M. F., Butcher, J. N., and Ben-Porath, Y. S. (1991). M.M.P.I.-2 profiles of women at risk for child abuse. *Journal of Personality Assessment, 57*(2), 254-263.

Egeland, B., Jacobvitz, D., and Sroufe, L. A. (1988). Breaking the cycle of abuse. *Child Development, 59*(4), 1080-1088.

Egeland, B., Weinfield, N. S., Bosquet, M., and Cheng, V. K. (2000). Remembering, repeating, and working through: Lessons from attachment-based interventions. In J. D. Osofsky and H. E. Fitzgerald (Eds.), *WAIMH Handbook of Infant Mental Health.* Vol. 4, *Infant Mental Health in Groups at High Risk* (pp. 35-89). New York: John Wiley and Sons, Inc.

Egley, L. C. (1991). What changes the societal prevalence of domestic violence? *Journal of Marriage and the Family, 53*(November), 885-897.

Emery, R. E. and Laumann-Billings, L. (1998). An overview of the nature, causes, and consequences of abusive family relationships: Toward differentiating maltreatment and violence. *American Psychologist, 53*(2), 121-135.

English, D. J. and Marshall, D. B. (1998). Risk assessment and CPS decision making. In J. Fluke, R. Alsop, and C. Race (Eds.), *Twelfth national roundtable on child protective services risk assessment: Summary of proceedings* (pp. 123-130). Englewood, CO: American Humane Association.

English, D. J., Marshall, D. B., Brummel, S., and Orme, M. (1999). Characteristics of repeated referrals to child protective services in Washington State. *Child Maltreatment, 4*(4), 297-307.

English, D. J. and Pecora, P. J. (1994). Risk assessment as a practice method in child protective services. *Child Welfare League of America, LXXII*(5), 451-473.

Erickson, M. F., and Egeland, B. (1996). Child neglect. In J. Myers, L. Berliner, J. Briere, J. C. T. Hendrix, C. Jenny, and T. Reid (Eds.), *The APSAC handbook on child maltreatment,* Second edition (pp. 3-20). Thousand Oaks, CA: Sage Publications.

Erickson, M. F. and Egeland, B. (2002). Child neglect. In J. Briere, L. Berliner, J. A. Bulkley, C. Jenny, and T. Reid (Eds.), *The APSAC handbook on child maltreatment,* Second edition (pp. 3-20). Thousand Oaks, CA: Sage Publications.

Everson, M. D., Hunter, W. M., Runyon, D. K., Edelsohn, G. A., and Coulter, M. L. (1989). Maternal support following disclosure of incest. *American Journal of Orthopsychiatry,* 59(2), 197-207.

Fahlberg, V. (1997, May). "Children's attachment issues." Maine Judicial Symposium on Decision-making in Permanency Planning, Newry, Maine.

Fantuzzo, J. W., DePaola, L. M., Lambert, L., Martino, T., Anderson, G., and Sutton, S. (1991). Effects of interparental violence on the psychological adjustment and competencies of young children. *Journal of Consulting and Clinical Psychology,* 59(2), 258-265.

Fehrenbach, P. A., Smith, W. R., Monastersky, C., and Deischer, R. W. (1986). Adolescent sexual offenders: Offender and offense characteristics. *Journal of Orthopsychiatry,* 56(2), 225-233.

Feiring, C., Taska, L. S., and Lewis, M. (1998). Social support and children's and adolescents' adaptations to sexual abuse. *Journal of Interpersonal Violence,* 13(2), 240-260.

Figley, C. R. (Ed.) (1995). *Compassion fatigue: Coping with secondary traumatic stress in those who treat the traumatized.* New York: Brunner/Mazel, Inc.

Findlater, J. E. and Kelly, S. (1999). Reframing child safety in Michigan: Building collaboration among domestic violence, family preservation, and child protection services. *Child Maltreatment,* 4(2), 167-174.

Finkelhor, D. (1997). The victimization of children and youth: Developmental victimology. In R. C. Davis, A. J. Lurigio, and W. G. Skogan (Eds.), *Victims of Crime,* Second edition (pp. 86-107). Thousand Oaks, CA: Sage Publications, Inc.

Finkelhor, D. and Berliner, L. (1995). Research on the treatment of sexually abused children: A review and recommendations. *Journal of the American Academy of Child and Adolescent Psychiatry,* 34(11), 1408-1423.

Firestone, P., Bradford, J. M., McCoy, M., Greenberg, D. M., Larose, M. R., Curry, S. (1999). Prediction of recidivism in incest offenders. *Journal of Interpersonal Violence,* 14(5), 511-531.

Fisher, P.A., Ellis, B., and Chamberlain, P. (1999). Early intervention foster care: A model for preventing risk in young children who have been maltreated. *Children's Services: Social Policy, Research, and Practice,* 2(3), 159-182.

Fluke, J., Edwards, M., Bussey, M., Wells, S., and Johnson, W. (2001). Reducing recurrence in child protective services: Impact of a targeted safety protocol. *Child Maltreatment,* 6(3), 207-218.

Fonagy, P., Leigh, T., Steele, M., Steele, H., Kennedy, R., Mattoon, G., Target, M., and Gerber, A. (1996). The relations of attachment status, psychiatric classification, and response to psychotherapy. *Journal of Consulting and Clinical Psychology, 64*(1), 22-31.

Forth, A. E. (1995). *Psychopathy and young offenders: Prevalence, family background, and violence.* Unpublished report, Carleton University, Ottawa, Ontario.

Forth, A. E., Hart, S. D., and Hare, R. D. (1990). Assessment of psychopathy in male young offenders. *Psychological Assessment: A Journal of Consulting and Clinical Psychology, 2*(3), 342-344.

Friedrich, W. N. (1990). *Psychotherapy of sexually abused children and their families.* New York: W. W. Norton and Company.

Friedrich, W. N. (1993). Sexual victimization and sexual behavior in children: A review of recent literature. *Child Abuse and Neglect, 17*(1), 59-66.

Friedrich, W. N. (1996). Clinical considerations of empirical treatment studies of abused children. *Child Maltreatment, 1*(4), 343-347.

Friedrich, W. N. (1997). *Child Sexual Behavior Inventory.* Odessa, FL: Psychological Assessment Resources.

Friedrich, W. N., Fisher, J., Broughton, D., Houston, M., and Shafran, C. (1998). Normative sexual behavior in children: a contemporary sample. *Pediatrics, 101*(4), 1-8.

Friedrich, W. N., Grambsch, P., Broughton, D., Kuiper, J., and Beilke, R. L. (1991). Normative sexual behavior in children. *Pediatrics, 88*(3), 456-464.

Friedrich, W. N., Grambsch, P., Damon, L., Hewitt, S. K., Koverola, C., Lang, R. A., Wolfe, V., and Broughton, D. (1992). Child Sexual Behavior Inventory: Normative and clinical comparisons. *Psychological Assessment, 4*(3), 303-311.

Friedrich, W. N., Tyler, J. D., and Clark, J. A. (1985). Personality and psychophysiological variables in abusive, neglectful, and low-income control mothers. *The Journal of Nervous and Mental Disease, 178*(8), 449-460.

Frodi, A. M., and Lamb, M. E. (1980). Child abusers' responses to infant smiles and cries. *Child Development, 51*, 238-241.

Frye v. United States, 293 F. 1013 (1923).

Fryer, G. E., Jr. and Miyoshi, T. J. (1996). The role of the environment in the etiology of child maltreatment. *Aggression and Violent Behavior, 1*(4), 317-326.

Gabinet, L. (1983). Child abuse treatment failures reveal need for redefinition of the problem. *Child Abuse and Neglect, 7*(4), 395-402.

Gacono, C. B. and Hutton, H. E. (1994). Suggestions for the clinical and forensic use of the Hare Psychopathy Checklist-Revised (PCL-R). *International Journal of Law and Psychiatry, 17*(3), 303-317.

Ganley, A. L. and Harris, L. (1978). *Domestic violence: Issues in designing and implementing programs for male batterers.* Paper presented at the meeting of the American Psychological Association, Toronto, August.

Garbarino, J. (1997). The role of economic deprivation in the social context of child maltreatment. In M. E. Helfer, R. S. Kempe, and R. D. Krugman (Eds.), *The battered child,* Fifth edition (pp. 49-60). Chicago: The University of Chicago Press.

Garbarino, J. and Kostelny, K. (1992). Child maltreatment as a community problem. *Child Abuse and Neglect, 16*(4), 455-464.

Gaudin, J. (1993). Effective interventions with neglectful families. *Criminal Justice and Behavior, 20*(1), 66-89.

Gaudin, J. (1999). Child neglect: Short-term and long-term outcomes. In H. Dubowitz (Ed.), *Neglected children: Research, practice, and policy* (pp. 89-108). Thousand Oaks, CA: Sage Publications.

Geffner, R. A. (1996). Editor's comment: Definitions of FV and use of terms. *Family Violence and Sexual Assault Bulletin, 12*(3-4), p3.

Gelles, R. (1996, September). "Children first: How to help child protective services assure child safety." Symposium conducted at the First Annual Northern New England Conference on Child Maltreatment, Portland, ME.

Gendreau, P., Little, T., and Goggin, C. (1996). A meta-analysis of the predictors of adult offender recidivism: What works! *Criminology, 34*(4), 401-433.

Gershater-Molko, R. M., Lutzker, J. R., and Wesch, D. (2002). Using recidivism data to evaluate Project SafeCare: Teaching bonding, safety, and health care skills to parents. *Child Maltreatment, 7*(3), 277-285.

Glaser, D. (2000). Child abuse and neglect and the brain: A review. *Journal of Child Psychology and Psychiatry and Allied Disciplines, 41*(1), 97-116.

Goldman, S. K. (1999). The conceptual framework for Wraparound: Definitions, values, essential elements, and requirements for practice. In B. J. Burns and S. K. Goldman (Eds.), *Systems of Care: Promising Practices in Children's Mental Health, 1998 Series.* Vol. IV. *Promising practices in wraparound for children with serious emotional disturbance and their families* (pp. 9-16). Washington, DC: Center for Effective Collaboration and Practice, American Institutes for Research.

Gomes-Schwartz, B., Horwitz, J. M., Cardarelli, A. P., Sauzier, M., Salt, P., and Calhoon, R. (1990). The effects of sexual abuse. In B. Schwartz, J. M. Horwitz, and A. P. Cardarelli (Eds.), *Child sexual abuse: The initial effects* (pp. 75-108). Newbury Park, CA: Sage Publications, Inc.

Gondolf, E. W. (1987). Changing men who batter: A developmental model for integrated interventions. *Journal of Family Violence, 2*(4), 335-349.

Gondolf, E. W. (1993). Male batterers. In R. L. Hampton, T. P Gullotta, G. R. Adams, E. H. Potter III, and R. P. Weissberg (Eds.), *Issues in children's and families' lives. Family violence prevention and treatment.* Vol. 1 (pp. 230-257). Newbury Park, CA: Sage Publications.

Gondolf, E. W. (1999). A comparison of four batterer intervention systems: Do court referral, program length, and services matter? *Journal of Interpersonal Violence, 14*(1), 41-61.

Goodman, S. H. and Brumley, H. E. (1990). Schizophrenic and depressed mothers: Relational deficits in parenting. *Developmental Psychology, 26*(1), 31-39.

Graham-Bermann, S. A., Cutler, S. E., Litzsenberger, B. W., and Schwartz, W. E. (1994). Perceived conflict and violence in childhood sibling relationships and later emotional adjustment. *Journal of Family Psychology, 8*, 85-97.

Gray, A. S., Busconi, A., Houchens, P., and Pithers, W. (1997). Children with sexual behavior problems and their caregivers: Demographics, functioning, and clinical patterns. *Sexual Abuse: A Journal of Research and Treatment, 9*(4), 267-290.

Gray, A. S. and Pithers, W. D. (1993). Relapse prevention with sexually aggressive adolescents and children: Expanding treatment and supervision. In H. E. Barbaree, W. L. Marshall, and S. M. Hudson (Eds.), *The juvenile sex offender* (pp. 289-319). New York: The Guilford Press.

Gray, J. D., Cutler, G. A., Dean, J. G., and Kempe, C. H. (1979). Prediction and prevention of child abuse and neglect. *Journal of Social Issues, 35*(2), 127-139.

Grayson, J. (1995). Treatment outcome for families who abuse or neglect. *Virginia Child Protection Newsletter, 46,* 8-16.

Grayson, J. (1996). Treatment outcome for spouses who batter. *Virginia Child Protection Newsletter, 50,* 1, 3-6, 12, 14, 15.

Greenberg, D. M. and Bradford, J. M. W. (1997). Treatment of the paraphilic disorders: A review of the role of the selective serotonin reuptake inhibitors. *Sexual Abuse: A Journal of Research and Treatment, 9*(4), 349-360.

Greenberg, M. T. and Speltz, M. L. (1988). Attachment and the ontogeny of conduct problems. In J. Belsky and T. Nezworski (Eds.), *Clinical Implications of Attachment* (pp. 177-218). Hillsdale, NJ: Lawrence Erlbaum Associates.

Griffiths, D. M., Quinsey, V. L., and Hingsburger, D. (1989). *Changing inappropriate sexual behavior: A community-based approach for persons with developmental disabilities.* Baltimore, MD: Paul H. Brookes.

Grisso, T. (1986). *Evaluating competencies. Forensic assessment and instruments.* New York: Plenum Press.

Grisso, T. (1998). *Forensic evaluation of juveniles.* Sarasota, FL: Professional Resource Press.

Grisso, T. and Applebaum, P. (1992). Is it unethical to offer predictions of future violence? *Law and Human Behavior, 16*(6), 621-633.

Grizenko, N. and Pawliuk, N. (1994). Risk and protective factors for disruptive behavior disorders in children. *American Journal of Orthopsychiatry, 64*(4), 534-544.

Grossman, L. S., Martis, B., and Fichtner, C. G. (1999). Are sex offenders treatable? A research overview. *Psychiatric Services, 50*(3), 349-361.

Hall, G. C. N. (1995). Sexual offender recidivism revisited: A meta-analysis of recent treatment studies. *Journal of Consulting and Clinical Psychology, 63*(5), 802-809.

Hall, G. C. N., Bansal, A., Lopez, E. (1999). Ethnicity and psychopathology: A meta-analytic review of 31 years of comparative MMPI/MMPI-2 research. *Psychological Assessment, 11*(2), 186-197.

Hall, G. C. N., Shondrick, D. D., and Hirschman, R. (1993). Conceptually derived treatments for sexual aggressors. *Professional Psychology: Research and Practice, 24*(1), 62-69.

Hansen, D. J. and Warner, J. E. (1994). Treatment adherence of maltreating families: A survey of professionals regarding prevalence and enhancement strategies. *Journal of Family Violence, 9*(1), 1-19.

Hansen, D. J., Warner-Rogers, J. E., and Hecht, D. B. (1998). Implementing and evaluating an individualized behavioral intervention program for maltreating families: Clinical and research issues. In J. R. Lutzker (Ed.), *Handbook of child abuse research and treatment* (pp. 133-158). New York: Plenum Press.

Hanson, R. K. (1996). Evaluating the contribution of relapse prevention theory to the treatment of sexual offenders. *Sexual Abuse: A Journal of Research and Treatment, 8*(3), 201-208.

Hanson, R. K. and Bussière, M. T. (1996). *Predictors of sexual offender recidivism: A meta-analysis.* Ottawa, Ontario, Canada: Public Works and Government Services.

Hanson, R. K. and Bussière, M. T. (1998). Predicting relapse: A meta-analysis of sexual offender recidivism studies. *Journal of Consulting and Clinical Psychology, 66*(2), 348-362.

Hanson, R. K. and Harris, A. J. (2000). Where should we intervene? Dynamic predictors of sex offense recidivism. *Criminal Justice and Behavior, 27*(1), 6-35.

Hanson, R. K. and Scott, H. (1996). Social networks of sexual offenders. *Psychology, Crime and Law, 2,* 249-258.

Hanson, R. K. and Thornton, D. (2000). Improving risk assessments for sex offenders: A comparison of three actuarial scales. *Law and Human Behavior, 24*(1), 119-136.

Hare, R. D. (1991). *Manual for the Hare Psychopathy Checklist-Revised.* North Tonawanda, NY: Multi-Health Systems.

Hare, R. D. (1996). Psychopathy: A clinical construct whose time has come. *Criminal Justice and Behavior, 23*(1), 25-54.

Hare, R. D., McPherson, L. E., and Forth, A. E. (1988). Male psychopaths and their criminal careers. *Journal of Consulting and Clinical Psychology, 56*(5), 710-714.

Harris, G. T., Rice, M. E., and Cormier, C. A. (1991). Psychopathy and violent recidivism. *Law and Human Behavior, 15*(6), 625-637.

Harris, G. T., Rice, M. E., and Quinsey, V. L. (1993). Violent recidivism of mentally disordered offenders: The development of a statistical prediction instrument. *Criminal Justice and Behavior, 20*(4), 315-355.

Hart, S. N., Brassard, M. R., Binggeli, N. J., Davidson, H. A. (2002). Psychological maltreatment. In J. Myers, L. Berliner, J. Briere, J. C. T. Hendrix, C. Jenny, and T. Reid (Eds.), *The APSAC handbook on child maltreatment* (pp. 79-104). Thousand Oaks, CA: Sage Publications.

Hart, S. N., Brassard, M. R., and Karlson, H. C. (1996). Psychological maltreatment. In J. Briere, L. Berliner, J. A. Bulkley, C. Jenny, and T. Reid (Eds.), *The APSAC handbook on child maltreatment* (pp. 72-89). Thousand Oaks, CA: Sage Publications.

Hart, S. D., Kropp, P. R., and Hare, R. D. (1988). Performance of psychopaths following conditional release from prison. *Journal of Consulting and Clinical Psychology, 56*(2), 227-232.

Hawkins, J. D., Herrenkohl, T., Farrington, D. P., Brewer, D., Catalano, R. F., and Harachi, T. W. (1998). A review of predictors of youth violence. In R. Loeber and D. P. Farrington (Eds.), *Serious and violent juvenile offenders: Risk factors and successful interventions* (pp. 106-146). Thousand Oaks, CA: Sage Publications.

Heilbrun, K. (1992). The role of psychological testing in forensic assessment. *Law and Human Behavior, 16*(3), 257-633.

Heinze, M. C. and Grisso, T. (1996). Review of instruments assessing parenting competencies used in child custody evaluations. *Behavioral Science and the Law, 14*(3), 293-313.

Henggeler, S. W., Schoenwald, S. K., Bourduin, C. M., Rowland, M. D., and Cunningham, P. E. (1998). *Multisystemic treatment of antisocial behavior in children and adolescents.* New York: The Guilford Press.

Henning, K., Leitenberg, H., Coffey, P., Turner, T., and Bennett, R. T. (1996). Long-term psychological and social impact of witnessing physical conflict between parents. *Journal of Interpersonal Violence, 11*(1), 35-51.

Herman, J. (1981). *Father-daughter incest.* Cambridge, MA: Harvard University Press.

Herrenkohl, E.C., Herrenkohl, R.C., and Egolf, B. (1994). Resilient early school-age children from maltreating homes: Outcomes in late adolescence. *American Journal of Orthopsychiatry, 64*(2), 301-309.

Herrenkohl, R. C., Herrenkohl, E. C., Egolf, B. P., and Wu, P. (1991). The developmental consequences of child abuse: The Lehigh Longitudinal Study. In R. H. Starr Jr. and D. A. Wolfe (Eds.). *The effects of child abuse and neglect: Issues and research.* New York: The Guilford Press.

Herzberger, S. D. and Tennen, H. (1985). "Snips and snails and puppy dog tails": Gender of agent, recipient, and observers as determinants of perceptions of discipline. *Sex Roles, 12*(7/8), 853-865.

Hess, P. M. and Folaron, G. (1991). Ambivalence: A challenge to permanency for children. *Child Welfare League of America, LXX*(4), 403-424.

Hess, P. M., Folaron, G., and Jefferson, A. B. (1992). Effectiveness of family reunification services: An innovative evaluative model. *Social Work, 37*(4), 304-311.

Hill, C. D., Rogers, R., and Bickford, M. E. (1996). Predicting aggressive and socially disruptive behavior in a maximum security forensic psychiatric hospital. *Journal of Forensic Sciences, 41*(1), 56-59.

Hillson, J. M. and Kuiper, N. (1994). Stress and coping model of child maltreatment. *Clinical Psychology Review, 14*(4), 261-285.

Holtzworth-Munroe, A. and Stuart, G. (1994). Typologies of male batterers: Three subtypes and the differences among them. *Psychological Bulletin, 116*(3), 476-497.

Hudson, S. M. and Ward, T. (1996). Introduction to the special issue on relapse prevention. *Sexual Abuse: A Journal of Research and Treatment, 8*(3), 173-175.

Hughes, D. A. (1997). *Facilitating developmental attachment: The road to emotional recovery and behavioral change in foster and adopted children.* Northvale, NJ: Jason Aronson Inc.

Hunter, J. A. Jr. and Becker, J. V. (1994). The role of deviant sexual arousal in juvenile sexual offending: Etiology, evaluation, and treatment. *Criminal Justice and Behavior, 21*(1), 132-149.

Hunter, J. A. Jr. and Figueredo, A. J. (1999). Factors associated with treatment compliance in a population of juvenile sexual offenders. *Sexual Abuse: A Journal of Research and Treatment, 11*(1), 49-67.

Hunter, J. A. Jr. and Lexier, L. J. (1998). Ethical and legal issues in the assessment and treatment of juvenile sex offenders. *Child Maltreatment, 3*(4), 339-348.

Irueste-Montes, A. M. and Montes, F. (1988). Court-ordered vs. voluntary treatment of abusive and neglectful parents. *Child Abuse and Neglect, 12*(1), 33-39.

Iwaniec, D. (1995). *The emotionally abused and neglected child: Identification, assessment and intervention.* New York: John Wiley and Sons.

Jacobs, W. L., Kennedy, W. A., and Meyer, J. B. (1997). Juvenile delinquents: A between-group comparison study of sexual and nonsexual offenders. *Sexual Abuse: A Journal of Research and Treatment, 9*(3), 201-218.

Jacobvitz, D. and Hazen, N. (1999). Developmental pathways from infant disorganization to childhood peer relationships. In J. Solomon and C. George (Eds.), *Attachment disorganization* (pp. 127-159). New York: The Guilford Press.

Jaffe, P. G. and Geffner, R. (1998). Child custody disputes and domestic violence: Critical issues for mental health, social services, and legal professionals. In G. W. Holden, R. Geffner, and E. N. Jouriles (Eds.), *Children exposed to marital violence: Theory, research, and applied issues* (pp. 371-408). Washington, DC: American Psychological Association.

Jaffe, P. G., Sudermann, M., and Reitzel, D. (1992). Child witnesses of marital violence. In R. Ammerman and M. Hersen (Eds.), *Assessment of family violence: A clinical and legal sourcebook* (pp. 313-331). New York: John Wiley and Sons.

Jaffe, P. G., Wilson, S. K., and Wolfe, D. A. (1988). Specific assessment and intervention strategies for children exposed to wife battering: Preliminary empirical investigations. *Canadian Journal of Community Mental Health, 7*(2), 157-163.

Jaffe, P. G., Wolfe, D. A., and Wilson, S. K. (1990). *Children of battered women.* Vol. 21, *Developmental Clinical Psychology and Psychiatry.* Newbury Park: Sage Publications.

Jaffe, P. G., Wolfe, D. A., Wilson, S. K., and Zak, L. (1986). Similarities in behavioral and social maladjustment among child victims and witnesses to family violence. *American Journal of Orthopsychiatry, 56*(1), 142-146.

Johnson, J. G., Cohen, P., Brown, J., Smailes, E. M., and Bernstein, D. P. (1999). Childhood maltreatment increases risk for personality disorders during early adulthood. *Archives of General Psychiatry, 56*(7), 600-606.

Johnson, W. B. (1988). Child-abusing parents: Factors associated with successful completion of treatment. *Psychological Reports, 63*(2), 434.

Jones, D. P. H. (1987). The untreatable family. *Child Abuse and Neglect, 11*(3), 409-420.

Jouriles, E. N. and Norwood, W. D. (1995). Physical aggression toward boys and girls in families characterized by the battering of women. *Journal of Family Psychology, 9,* 69-78.

Kafka, M. P. (1997). A monoamine hypothesis for the pathophysiology of paraphilic disorders. *Archives of Sexual Behavior, 26*(4), 343-358.

Kahn, T. J. and Chambers, H. J. (1991). Assessing reoffense risk with juvenile sexual offenders. *Child Welfare, LXX*(3), 333-345.

Kalichman, S., Henderson, M. C., Shealy, L. S., and Dwyer, M. (1992). Psychometric properties of the Multiphasic Sex Inventory in assessing sex offenders. *Criminal Justice and Behavior, 19*(4), 384-396.

Kamradt, B. (2000). Wraparound Milwaukee: Aiding youth with mental health needs. *Juvenile Justice Journal, VII*(1), 14-23.

Kandel-Englander, E. (1992). Wife battering and violence outside the family. *Journal of Interpersonal Violence, 7*(4), 462-270.

Kaufman, J. (1991). Depressive disorders in maltreated children. *Journal of the American Academy of Child and Adolescent Psychiatry, 30*(2), 257-265.

Kaufman, K. L. and Rudy, L. (1991). Future directions in the treatment of physical child abuse. *Criminal Justice and Behavior, 18*(1), 82-97.

Kavoussi, R. J., Kaplan, M., and Becker, J. V. (1988). Psychiatric diagnoses in adolescent sex offenders. *Journal of the American Academy of Child and Adolescent Psychiatry, 27*(2), 241-243.

Kear-Colwell, J. and Pollock, P. (1997). Motivation or confrontation: Which approach to the child sex offender? *Criminal Justice and Behavior, 24*(1), 20-33.

Kelleher, K., Chaffin, M., Hollenberger, J., and Fischer, E. (1994). Alcohol and drug disorders among physically abusive and neglectful parents in a community-based sample. *The American Journal of Public Health, 84*(10), 1586-1590.

Kendall-Tackett, K. A., Williams, L. M., and Finkelhor, D. (1993). Impact of sexual abuse in children: A review and synthesis of recent empirical studies. *Psychological Bulletin, 113*(1), 164-180.

Klassen, D. and O'Connor, W. A. (1988). A prospective study of predictors of violence in adult male mental health admissions. *Law and Human Behavior, 12*(2), 143-158.

Klassen, D. and O'Connor, W. A. (1994). Demographic and case history variables. In J. Monahan and H. J. Steadman (Eds.), *Violence and mental disorder: Developments in risk assessment* (pp. 229-257). Chicago: University of Chicago Press.

Knight, K. W. and Tripodi, T. (1996). Societal bonding and delinquency: An empirical test of Hirschi's theory of control. *Journal of Offender Rehabilitation, 23*(1-2), 117-129.

Knight, R. A. (1992). The generation and corroboration of a taxonomic model for child molesters. In W. O'Donohue and J. H. Geer (Eds.), *The sexual abuse of children: Clinical Issues.* Vol. 2 (pp. 24-70). Hillsdale, NJ: Lawrence Erlbaum Associates.

Knight, R. A. and Prentky, R. A. (1990). Classifying sexual offenders: The development and corroboration of taxonomic models. In W. L. Marshall, D. R. Laws, and H. E. Barbaree (Eds.), *The handbook of sexual assault: Issues, theories, and treatment of the offender* (pp. 27-52). New York: Plenum Press.

Knutson, J. J. (1995). Psychological characteristics of maltreated children: Putative risk factors and consequences. *Annual Review of Psychology, 46,* 401-431.

Kobayashi, J., Sales, B. D., Becker, J. V., Figueredo, A. J., and Kaplan, M. S. (1995). Perceived parental deviance, parent-child bonding, child abuse, and child sexual aggression. *Sexual Abuse: A Journal of Research and Treatment, 7*(1), 25-44.

Kolbo, J. R., Blakely, E. H., and Engleman, D. (1996). Children who witness domestic violence: A review of empirical literature. *Journal of Interpersonal Violence, 11*(2), 281-293.

Kolko, D. J. (1992). Characteristics of child victims of physical violence: Research findings and clinical implications. *Journal of Interpersonal Violence, 7*(2), 244-276.

Kolko, D. J. (1996). Individual cognitive behavioral treatment and family therapy for physically abused children and their offending parents: A comparison of clinical outcomes. *Child Maltreatment, 1*(4), 322-342.

Kolko, D. J. (1998). Treatment and intervention for child victims of violence. In P. K. Trickett and C. J. Schellenbach (Eds.), *Violence against children in the family and the community* (pp. 213-249). Washington, DC: American Psychological Association.

Kolko, D. J. (2002). Child physical abuse. In J. Briere, L. Berliner, J. A. Bulkley, C. Jenny, and T. Reid (Eds.), *The APSAC handbook on child maltreatment,* Second edition, (pp. 21-54). Thousand Oaks, CA: Sage Publications.

Kolko, D. J. (2002). Child physical abuse. In J. Myers, L. Berliner, J. Briere, J. C. T. Hendrix, C. Jenny, and T. Reid (Eds.), *The APSAC handbook on child maltreatment,* Second edition (pp. 21-54). Thousand Oaks, CA: Sage Publications.

Kropp, P. R., Hart, S. D., Webster, C. D., and Eaves, D. (1995). *Manual for the spousal assault risk assessment guide,* Second edition. Vancouver, British Columbia, Canada: The British Columbia Institute on Family Violence.

Kuehnle, K. (1996). *Assessing allegations of child sexual abuse.* Sarasota, FL: Professional Resource Press.

Kuehnle, K. (1998). Ethics and the forensic expert: A case study of child custody involving allegations of child sexual abuse. *Ethics and Behavior, 8*(1), 1-18.

Kwan, K. K. (1999). MMPI and MMPI-2 performance of the Chinese: Cross-cultural applicability. *Professional Psychology: Research and Practice, 30*(3), 260-268.

Lab, S., Shields, G., and Schondel, C. (1993). Research note: An evaluation of juvenile sexual offender treatment. *Crime and Delinquency, 39*(4), 543-553.

Langevin, R., Hucker, S. J., Handy, L., Purins, J. E., Russon, A. E., and Hook, H. J. (1985). Erotic preference and aggression in pedophilia: A comparison of heterosexual, homosexual, and bisexual types. In R. Langevin (Ed.), *Erotic preference, gender identity and aggression in men: New research studies* (pp. 137-160). Hillsdale, NJ: Lawrence Erlbaum Associates.

Langevin, R., Lang, R. A., and Curnoe, S. (1998). The prevalence of sex offenders with deviant fantasies. *Journal of Interpersonal Violence, 13*(3), 315-327.

Langevin, R. and Watson, R. J. (1996). Major factors in the assessment of paraphilics and sex offenders. *Journal of Offender Rehabilitation, 23*(3-4), (Special issue: Sex Offender Treatment: Biological Dysfunction, Intrapsychic Conflict, Interpersonal Violence), 39-70.

Levesque, R. J. R. (2000). Cultural evidence, child maltreatment, and the law. *Child Maltreatment, 5*(2), 146-160.

Limandri, B. J. and Seridan, D. J. (1995). Prediction of intentional interpersonal violence: An introduction. In J. C. Campbell (Ed.), *Assessing dangerousness: Violence by sexual offenders, batterers, and child abusers* (pp. 1-19). Thousand Oaks, CA: Sage Publications.

Link, B. G. and Stueve, A. (1994). Psychotic symptoms and the violent/illegal behavior of mental patients compared to community controls. In J. Monahan and H. J. Steadman (Eds.), *Violence and mental disorder: Developments in risk assessment* (pp. 137-159). Chicago: University of Chicago Press.

Lisak, D. and Ivan, C. (1995). Deficits in intimacy and empathy in sexually aggressive men. *Journal of Interpersonal Violence, 10*(3) 296-308.

Lizardi, H., Klein, D. N., Ouimette, P. C., Riso, L. P., Anderson, R. L., and Donaldson, S. K. (1995). Reports of childhood home environment in early-onset dysthymia and episodic major depression. *Journal of Abnormal Psychology, 104*(1), 132-139.

Looney, J. G. (1984). Treatment planning in child psychiatry. *Journal of the American Academy of Child Psychiatry, 23*(5), 529-536.

Lowry, R., Sleet, D., Duncan, C., Powell, K., and Kolbe, L. (1995). Adolescents at risk for violence. *Educational Psychology Review, 7*(1), 7-39.

Lundquist, L. M. and Hansen, D. J. (1998). Enhancing treatment adherence, social validity, and generalization of parent-training interventions with physically abusive and neglectful families. In J. R. Lutzker (Ed.), *Handbook of child abuse research and treatment* (pp. 449-471). New York: Plenum Press.

Lutzker, J. R. (Ed.) (1998). *Handbook of child abuse research and treatment.* New York: Plenum Press.

Lutzker, J. R., Bigelow, K. M., Doctor, R. M., Gershater, R. M., and Greene, B. F. (1998). An ecobehavioral model for the prevention and treatment of child abuse and neglect: History and applications. In J. R. Lutzker (Ed.), *Handbook of child abuse research and treatment* (pp. 239-266). New York: Plenum Press.

Lynch, M. and Cicchetti, D. (1991). Patterns of relatedness in maltreated and nonmaltreated children: Connections among multiple representational models. *Development and Psychopathology, 3*(2), 207-226.

Lyons, E. (1993). Hospital staff reactions to accounts by survivors of childhood abuse. *American Journal of Orthopsychiatry, 63*(3), 410-416.

Lyons-Ruth, K. (1996). Attachment relationships among children with aggressive behavior problems: The role of disorganized early attachment patterns. *Journal of Consulting and Clinical Psychology, 64*(1), 64-73.

MacArthur Violence Risk Assessment Study. April 2001. Executive Summary. www.macarthur.virginia.edu/risk.html.

Magdol, L., Moffitt, T. E., Caspi, A., and Silva, P. A. (1998). Long-term predictors of partner abuse. *Journal of Abnormal Psychology, 107*(3), 375-389.

Main, M. and Solomon, J. (1990). Procedures for identifying infants as disorganized/disoriented during the Ainsworth Strange Situation. In M. T. Greenberg, D. Cicchetti, and E. M. Cummings (Eds.), *Attachment in the Preschool Years* (pp. 51-86). Chicago: University of Chicago Press.

Malamuth, N. M., Sockloskie, R. J., Koss, M. P., and Tanaka, J. S. (1991). Characteristics of aggressors against women: Testing a model using a national sample of college students. *Journal of Consulting and Clinical Psychology, 59*(5), 670-681.

Maletzky, B. M. (1999). Groups of one. *Sexual Abuse: A Journal of Research and Treatment, 11*(3), 179-181.

Malinosky-Rummell, R. and Hansen, D. (1993). Long-term consequences of childhood physical abuse. *Psychological Bulletin, 114*(1), 68-79.

Manly, J. T., Cicchetti, D., and Barnett, D. (1994). The impact of subtype, frequency, chronicity, and severity of child maltreatment on social competence and behavior problems. *Development and Psychopathology, 6,* 121-143.

Mannarino, A. P. and Cohen, J. A. (1996). A follow-up study of factors that mediate the development of psychological symptomatology in sexually abused girls. *Child Maltreatment, 1*(3), 246-260.

Margolin, L. (1990). Fatal child neglect. *Child Welfare, LXIX*(4), 309-319.

Marker, A. H., Kemmelmeier, M., and Peterson, C. (1999). Parental sociopathy as a predictor of childhood sexual abuse. *Journal of Family Violence, 14*(1), 47-59.

Marques, J.K. (1995, September). *How to answer the question: Does sex offender treatment work?* Paper presented at the International Expert Conference on Sex Offenders: Issues, Research and Treatment, Utrecht, The Netherlands.

Marshall, D. B. and English, D. J. (1999). Survival analysis of risk factors for recidivism in child abuse and neglect. *Child Maltreatment, 4*(4), 287-296.

Marshall, W. L. (1996). An evaluation of the benefits of relapse prevention programs with sexual offenders. *Sexual Abuse: A Journal of Research and Treatment, 8*(3), 209-222.

Marshall, W. L. and Barbaree, H. E. (1990). Outcome of comprehensive cognitive-behavioral treatment programs. In W. L. Marshall, D. R. Laws, and H. E.

Barbaree (Eds.), *Handbook of sexual assault: Issues, theories, and treatment of the offender* (pp. 363-385). New York: Plenum Press.

Marshall, W. L., Hudson, S. M., and Hodkinson, S. (1993). The importance of attachment bonds in the development of juvenile sex offending. In H. Barbaree, W. Marshall, and S. Hudson (Eds.), *The juvenile sex offender* (pp. 164-181). New York: The Guilford Press.

Marshall, W. L. and Maric, A. (1996). Cognitive and emotional components of generalized empathy deficits in child molesters. *Journal of Child and Sexual Abuse, 5*(2), 101-111.

Marshall, W. L. and Pithers, W. D. (1994). A reconsideration of treatment outcome with sex offenders. *Criminal Justice and Behavior, 21*(1), 10-27.

Marshall, W. L., Serran, G. A., and Cortoni, F. A. (2000). Childhood attachments, sexual abuse, and their relationship to adult coping in child molesters. *Sexual Abuse: A Journal of Research and Treatment, 12*(1), 17-26.

Mash, E. H. (1991). Measurement of parent-child interactions in studies of maltreatment. In R. H. Starr Jr. and D. A. Wolfe (Eds.), *The effects of child abuse and neglect* (pp. 203-256). New York: The Guilford Press.

McCann, J. T. (1998). *Malingering and deception in adolescents: Assessing credibility in clinical and forensic settings.* Washington, DC: American Psychological Association.

McCann, J. T. and Dyer, F. J. (1996). *Forensic assessment with the Millon inventories.* New York: The Guilford Press.

McConnell, D., Llewellyn, G., and Bye, R. (1997). Providing services for parents with intellectual disability: Parent needs and service constraints. *Journal of Intellectual and Developmental Disability, 22*(1), 5-17.

McGee, R. A., Wolfe, D. A., and Wilson, S. K. (1997). Multiple maltreatment experiences and adolescent behavior problems: Adolescents' perspectives. *Development and Psychopathology, 9*(1), 131-149.

McGee, R. A., Wolfe, D. A., Yuen, S. A., Wilson, S. K., and Carnochan, J. (1995). The measurement of maltreatment: A comparison of approaches. *Child Abuse and Neglect, 19*(2), 233-249.

McKay, M. M. (1994). The link between domestic violence and child abuse: Assessment and treatment considerations. *Child Welfare, LXXIII*(1), 29-39.

McMillen, C. and Zuravin, S. (1997). Attributions of blame and responsibility for child sexual abuse and adult adjustment. *Journal of Interpersonal Violence, 12*(1), 30-48.

Meezan, W. and O'Keefe, M. (1998). Evaluating the effectiveness of multifamily group therapy in child abuse and neglect. *Research on Social Work Practice, 8*(3), 330-353.

Melton, G. B., Petrila, J., Poythress, N. G., and Slobogin, C. (1987). *Psychological evaluations for the courts.* New York: The Guilford Press.

Melton, G. B., Petrila, J., Poythress, N. G., and Slobogin, C. (1997). *Psychological evaluations for the courts,* Second edition. New York: The Guilford Press.

Mennen, F. E. and Meadow, D. (1995). The relationship of abuse characteristics to symptoms in sexually abused girls. *Journal of Interpersonal Violence, 10*(3), 259-274.

Messman-Moore, T. L. and Long, P. J. (2000). Child sexual abuse and revictimization in the form of adult sexual abuse, adult physical abuse, and adult psychological maltreatment. *Journal of Interpersonal Violence, 15*(5), 489-502.

Meyer, B. L. and Wagner, D. (1998). Using actuarial risk assessment to identify unsubstantiated cases for preventative intervention in New Mexico. In J. Fluke, R. Alsop, and C. Race (Eds.), *Twelfth national roundtable on child protective services risk assessment: Summary of proceedings* (pp. 87-102). Englewood, CO: American Humane Association.

Meyers, J., Kaufman, M., and Goldman, S. (1999). Promising practices: Training strategies for serving children with serious emotional disturbance and their families in a system of care. *Systems of Care: Promising Practices in Children's Mental Health, 1998 Series.* Vol. V. Washington, DC: Center for Effective Collaboration and Practice, American Institutes for Research.

Mihalic, S., Irwin, K., Elliott, D., Fagan, A., and Hansen, D. (2001). *Blueprints for Violence Prevention.* Rockville, MD: U.S. Dept of Justice. Office of Juvenile Justice and Delinquency Prevention, July.

Miller, P. M. and Lisak, D. (1999). Associations between childhood abuse and personality disorder symptoms in college males. *Journal of Interpersonal Violence, 14*(6), 642-656.

Miller, S. H. (1984). The relationship between adolescent childbearing and child maltreatment. *Child Welfare, 63*(6), 553-557.

Miller, W. R., Brown, J. M., Simpson, T. L., Handmaker, M. S., Bien, T. H., Luckie, L. F., Montgomery, H. A., Hester, R. K., and Tonigan, J. S. (1995). What works? A methodological analysis of the alcohol treatment outcome literature. In W. R. Miller and R. K. Hester (Eds.), *Handbook of alcohol treatment approaches, effective alternatives,* Second edition (pp. 12-44). Boston: Allyn and Bacon.

Miller, W. R. and Rollnick, S. (1991). *Motivational interviewing: Preparing people to change addictive behavior.* New York: The Guilford Press.

Miller-Perrin, C. L. and Perrin, R. (1999). *Child Maltreatment: An Introduction.* Thousand Oaks, CA: Sage.

Milloy, C. D. (1994, June). *A comparative study of juvenile sex offenders and non-sex offenders.* Olympia, WA: Washington State Institute for Public Policy.

Milner, J. S. (1986). *The Child Abuse Potential Inventory.* DeKalb, IL: Psytec Inc.

Milner, J. S. (1993). Social information processing and physical child abuse. *Clinical Psychology Review, 13*(3), 275-294.

Milner, J. S. (1994). Assessing physical child abuse risk: The child abuse potential inventory. *Clinical Psychology Review, 14*(6), 547-583.

Milner, J. S. (1995). Physical child abuse assessment: Perpetrator evaluation. In J. C. Campbell (Ed.), *Assessing dangerousness: Violence by sexual offenders, batterers, and child abusers* (pp. 41-67). Thousand Oaks, CA: Sage Publications.

Milner, J. S. (1998). Individual and family characteristics associated with intrafamilial child physical and sexual abuse. In P. K. Trickett and C. J. Schellenbach (Eds.), *Violence against children in the family and the community* (pp. 141-170). Washington, DC: American Psychological Association.

Milner, J. S. and Campbell, J. C. (1995). Prediction issues for practitioners. In J. C. Campbell (Ed.), *Assessing dangerousness: Violence by sexual offenders, batterers, and child abusers* (pp. 20-40). Thousand Oaks, CA: Sage Publications.

Milner, J. S. and Chilamkurti, C. (1991). Physical child abuse perpetrator characteristics: A review of the literature. *Journal of Interpersonal Violence, 6*(3), 345-366.

Milner, J. S. and Crouch, J. L. (1993). Physical child abuse. In R. L. Hampton, T. P. Gullotta, G. A. Adams, E. H. Potter III, and R. P. Weissberg (Eds.), *Family violence prevention and treatment: Issues in children's and families' lives.* Vol. 1 (pp. 25-55). Newbury Park, CA: Sage Publications.

Milner, J. S. and Dopke, C. A. (1997). Child physical abuse: Review of offender characteristics. In D. A. Wolfe, R. J. McMahon, and R. D. Peters (Eds.), *Child abuse: New directions in prevention and treatment across the lifespan* (pp. 27-54). Thousand Oaks, CA: Sage Publications.

Milner, J. S. and McCanne, T. R. (1991). Neuropsychological correlates of physical child abuse. In J. S. Milner (Ed.), *Neuropsychology of Aggression* (pp. 131-145). Boston: Kluwer Academic.

Milner, J. S. and Murphy, W. D. (1995). Assessment of child physical and sexual abuse offenders. *Family Relations, 44*(4), 478-488.

Milner, J. S., Murphy, W. D., Valle, L. A., and Tolliver, R. M. (1998). Assessment issues in child abuse evaluations. In J. R. Lutzker (Ed.), *Handbook of child abuse research and treatment* (pp. 75-115). New York: Plenum Press.

Miner, M. H. and Crimmins, C. L. S. (1995). Adolescent sex offenders—Issues of etiology and risk factors. In B. K. Schwartz and H. K. Cellini (Eds.), *The sex offender.* Vol. II. *Corrections, treatment and legal practice.* (9-1 – 9-15). Kingston, NJ: Civic Research Institute.

Miner, M. H., Siekert, G. P., and Ackland, M. A. (1997). *Evaluation: Juvenile sex offender treatment program, Minnesota Correctional Facility – Sauk Centre* (Final report – Biennium 1995-1997). Minneapolis, MN: University of Minnesota, Department of Family Practice and Community Health, Program in Human Sexuality.

Monahan, J. (1981). *The clinical prediction of violent behavior.* Rockville, MD: U.S. Department of Health and Human Services, National Institute of Mental Health.

Monahan, J. (1993). Limiting therapist exposure to *Tarasoff* Liability: Guidelines for risk containment. *American Psychologist, 48*(3), 242-250.

Monahan, J. and Steadman, H. J. (1994). Toward a rejuvenation of risk assessment research. In J. Monahan and H. J. Steadman (Eds.), *Violence and mental disor-*

der: Developments in risk assessment (1-17). Chicago: University of Chicago Press.

Moncher, F. J. (1996). The relationship of maternal adult attachment style and risk of physical child abuse. *Journal of Interpersonal Violence, 11*(3), 335-350.

Moore, E., Armsden, G., and Gogerty, P. (1998). A twelve-year follow-up study of maltreated and at-risk children who received early therapeutic child care. *Child Maltreatment, 3*(1), 3-17.

Moore, T. D. (1998). Kansas initiative for decision support. In J. Fluke, R. Alsop, and C. Race (Eds.), *Twelfth national roundtable on child protective services risk assessment: Summary of proceedings* (pp. 17-36). Englewood, CO: American Humane Association.

Mosher, K. K. (1998). Treatment recommendations for the chaotic or multiproblem maltreating parent including parents with mental illness or mental retardation. *In the Forum, 3*(2), 8-9.

Mosher, K. K. and Righthand, S. C. (1995, June). Recommendations for mental health and risk assessment. In the *Report of Maine's Multidisciplinary Review Panel on Child Deaths and Serious Injuries Due to Abuse or Neglect.* Augusta, ME: Department of Human Services.

Moss, E., St-Laurent, D., and Parent, S. (1999). Disorganized attachment and developmental risk at school age. In J. Solomon and C. George (Eds.), *Attachment disorganization* (pp. 160-186). New York: The Guilford Press.

Mossman, D. (1994). Assessing predictions of violence: Being accurate about accuracy. *Journal of Consulting and Clinical Psychology, 62*(4), 783-792.

Mrazek, P. J. (1993). Maltreatment and infant development. In C. H. Zeanah Jr. (Ed.), *Handbook of Infant Mental Health* (pp. 159-170). New York: The Guilford Press.

Mullen, P. E., Martin, J. L., Anderson, J. C., Romans, S. E., and Herbison, G. P. (1996). The long-term impact of the physical, emotional, and sexual abuse of children: A community study. *Child Abuse and Neglect, 20*(1), 7-21.

Muller, R. T., Caldwell, R. A., and Hunter, J. E. (1993). Child provocativeness and gender as factors contributing to the blaming of victims of physical child abuse. *Child Abuse and Neglect, 17*(2), 249-260.

Murphy, J. M, Bishop, S. J., Jellinek, M. S., Quinn, D., and Poitrast, F. G. (1992). What happens after the care and protection petition? Reabuse in a court sample. *Child Abuse and Neglect, 16*(4), 485-493.

Murphy, W. D. and Smith, T. A. (1996). Sex offenders against children: Empirical and clinical issues. In J. Briere, L. Berliner, J. A. Bulkley, C. Jenny, and T. Reid (Eds.), *The APSAC handbook on child maltreatment* (pp. 4-20). Thousand Oaks, CA: Sage Publications.

Murphy-Berman, V. (1994). A conceptual framework for thinking about risk assessment and case management in child protective service. *Child Abuse and Neglect, 18*(2), 193-201.

National Adolescent Perpetrator Network (1993). The revised report from the National Task Force on Juvenile Sexual Offending. *Juvenile and Family Court Journal, 44*(4), 1-120.

National Council of Juvenile and Family Court Judges (1998). *Family violence: Emerging programs for battered mothers and their children.* October. Reno, Nevada: Author.

Nayak, M. and Milner, J. S. (1995). *Neuropsychological correlates of physical child abuse.* Unpublished manuscript.

Negy, C. and Snyder, D. K. (2000). Reliability and equivalence of the Spanish translation of the Marital Satisfaction Inventory-Revised (MSI-R). *Psychological Assessment, 12,* 425-430.

Nelson, K. E., Saunders, E. J., and Lansman, M. J. (1993). Chronic child neglect in perspective. *Social Work, 38*(2), 661-671.

Neumann, D. A., Houskamp, B. M., Pollock, V. E., and Briere, J. (1996). The long-term sequelae of childhood sexual abuse in women: A meta-analytic review. *Child Maltreatment, 1*(1), 6-16.

Newman, C. F. (1994). Understanding client resistance: Methods for enhancing motivation to change. *Cognitive and Behavioral Practice, 1*(1), 47-69.

Ney, P. G., Fung, T., and Wickett, A. R. (1994). The worst combinations of child abuse and neglect. *Child Abuse and Neglect, 18*(9), 705-714.

Nichols, H. R. and Molinder, I. (1984). *The Multiphasic Sex Inventory.* Tacoma, WA: Authors.

Nichols, H. R. and Molinder, I. (1996). *Multiphasic Sex Inventory-II.* Tacoma, WA: Authors.

Nuttall, R. and Jackson, H. (1994). Personal history of childhood abuse among clinicians. *Child Abuse and Neglect, 18*(5), 455-472.

Oates, M. (1997). Patients as parents: The risk to children. *British Journal of Psychiatry, 170*(32), 22-27.

Okazaki, S. and Sue, S. (2000). Implications of test revisions for assessment with Asian Americans. *Psychological Assessment, 12*(3), 272-280.

O'Keefe, M. (1994). Adjustment of children from maritally violent homes. *Families in Society: The Journal of Contemporary Human Services, 75*(7), 403-415.

O'Keefe, M. (1997). Predictors of dating violence among high school students. *Journal of Interpersonal Violence, 12*(4), 546-568.

Oldershaw, L., Walters, G. C., and Hall, D. K. (1986). Control strategies and non-compliance in abusive mother-child dyads: An observational study. *Child Development, 57*(3), 722-732.

O'Leary, D. (1996). Physical aggression in intimate relationships can be treated within a marital context under certain circumstances. *Journal of Interpersonal Violence, 11*(3), 450-452.

Pagelow, M.D. (1981). *Woman-battering: Victims and their experiences.* Beverly Hills, CA: Sage Publications.

Patterson, G. R. and Chamberlain, P. (1994). A functional analysis of resistance during parent training therapy. *Clinical Psychology: Science and Practice, 1*(1), 53-70.

Pearce, J. W. and Pezzot-Pearce, T. D. (1997). *Psychotherapy of abused and neglected children.* New York: The Guilford Press.

Perez, C. M. and Widom, C. S. (1994). Childhood victimization and long-term intellectual and academic outcomes. *Child Abuse and Neglect, 18*(8), 617-633.

Perrin, G. I. and Sales, B. D. (1994). Forensic standards in the American Psychological Association's new ethics code. *Professional Psychology: Research and Practice, 25*(4), 376-381.

Pianta, R., Egeland, B., and Erickson, M. F. (1989). The antecedents of maltreatment: Results of the Mother-Child Interaction Research Project. In D. Cicchetti and V. Carlson (Eds.), *Child maltreatment: Theory and research on the causes and consequences of child abuse and neglect* (pp. 203-253). New York: Cambridge University Press.

Pithers, W. D. (1999). Empathy: Definition, enhancement, and relevance to the treatment of sexual abusers. *Journal of Interpersonal Violence, 14*(3), 257-284.

Pithers, W. D., Gray, A., Busconi, A., and Houchens, P. (1998). Children with sexual behavior problems: Identification of five distinct child types and related treatment considerations. *Child Maltreatment, 3*(4), 384-406.

Pithers, W. D., Kashima, K. M., Cumming, G. F., Beal, L. S., and Buell, M. M. (1987). "Relapse prevention of sexual aggression." Paper presented at the meeting of the New York Academy of Sciences Human Sexual Aggression conference, New York, NY.

Pithers, W. D., Marques, J. K., Gibat, C. C., and Marlatt, G. A. (1993). Relapse prevention with sexual aggressives: A self-control model of treatment and maintenance of change. In J. G. Greer and I. S. Stuart (Eds.), *The sexual aggressor: Current perspectives on treatment* (pp. 214-239). New York: Van Nostrand Reinhold Company.

Polansky, N. A., Chalmers, M. A., Buttenweiser, E., and Williams, D. P. (1981). *Damaged parents: An anatomy of child neglect.* Chicago: The University of Chicago Press.

Poole, D. A. and Lamb, M. E. (1998). *Investigative interviews of children: A guide for helping professionals.* Washington, DC: American Psychological Association.

Preciado, J. and Henry, M. (1997). Linguistic barriers in health education and services. In J. C. García and M. C. Zea (Eds.), *Psychological Interventions and Research with Latino Populations* (pp. 235-254). Boston: Allyn and Bacon.

Prentky, R. A. (1997). Arousal reduction in sexual offenders: A review of antiandrogen interventions. *Sexual Abuse: A Journal of Research and Treatment, 9*(4), 335-347.

Prentky, R. A., Burgess, A. W., Rokous, G., Lee, A., Hartman, C., Ressler, R., and Douglas, J. (1989). The presumptive role of fantasy in serial sexual homicide. *American Journal of Psychiatry, 146*(7), 887-891.

Prentky, R. A. and Knight, R. A. (1986). Impulsivity in the lifestyle and criminal behavior of sexual offenders. *Criminal Justice and Behavior, 13*(2), 141-164.

Prentky, R. A. and Knight, R. A. (1993). Age of onset of sexual assault: Criminal and life history correlates. In G. C. Nagayama Hall, R. Hirschman, J. R. Graham, and M. S. Zaragoza (Eds.), *Sexual aggression: Issues in etiology, assessment, and treatment* (pp. 43-62). Washington, DC: Taylor and Francis.

Prentky, R. A., Knight, R. A., and Lee, A. F. S. (1997). Risk factors associated with recidivism among extrafamilial child molesters. *Journal of Consulting and Clinical Psychology, 65*(1), 141-149.

Prentky, R., and Righthand, S. (2001). *Juvenile sex offender assessment protocol: Manual.* Bridgewater, MA.

Prochaska, J. O., DiClemente, C. C., and Norcross, J. C. (1992). In search of how people change: Applications to addictive behaviors. *American Psychologist, 47*(9), 1102-1114.

Proulx, J., Cote, G., and Achille, P. A. (1993). Prevention of voluntary control of penile response in homosexual pedophiles during phallometric testing. *The Journal of Sex Research, 30*(2), 140-147.

Quinsey, V. L., Harris, G. T., Rice, M. E., and Cormier, C. A. (1998). *Violent offenders: Appraising and managing risk.* Washington, DC: American Psychological Association.

Quinsey, V. L., Harris, G. T., Rice, M. E., and Lalumière, M. L. (1993). Assessing treatment efficacy in outcome studies of sex offenders. *Journal of Interpersonal Violence, 8*(4), 512-523.

Quinsey, V. L. and Lalumière, M. L. (1996). *Assessment of sexual offenders against children: The APSAC study guides 1.* Thousand Oaks, CA: Sage Publications.

Quinsey, V. L., Lalumière, M. L., Rice, M. E., and Harris, G. T. (1995). Predicting sexual offenses. In J. C. Campbell (Ed.), *Assessing dangerousness: Violence by sexual offenders, batterers, and child abusers* (pp. 114-137). Thousand Oaks, CA: Sage Publications.

Quinsey, V. L., Reid, K. S., and Stermac, L. E. (1996). Mentally disordered offenders' accounts of their crimes. *Criminal Justice and Behavior, 23*(3), 472-489.

Quinsey, V. L., Rice, M. E., and Harris, G. T. (1995). Actuarial prediction of sexual recidivism. *Journal of Interpersonal Violence, 10*(1), 85-105.

Raine, A., Brennan, P., and Mednick, S. A. (1997). Interaction between birth complications and early maternal rejection in predisposing individuals to adult violence: Specificity to serious, early-onset violence. *American Journal of Psychiatry, 154*(9), 1265-1271.

Raine, A., Venables, P. H., and Williams, M. (1990). Relationships between central and autonomic measures of arousal at age 15 years and criminality at age 24 years. *Archives of General Psychiatry, 47*(11), 1003-1007.

Rasmussen, L. A. (1999). Factors related to recidivism among juvenile sexual offenders. *Sexual Abuse: A Journal of Research and Treatment, 11*(1), 69-85.

Ray, K. C. and Jackson, J. L. (1997). Family environment and childhood sexual victimization: A test of the buffering hypothesis. *Journal of Interpersonal Violence, 12*(1), 3-17.

Reeker, J., Ensing, D., and Elliot, R. (1997). A meta-analytic investigation of group treatment outcomes for sexually abused children. *Child Abuse and Neglect, 21*(7), 669-680.

Reiss Miller, L. P. and Azar, S. T. (1996, Fall/Winter). The pervasiveness of maladaptive attributions in mothers at risk for child abuse. *Family Violence and Sexual Assault Bulletin,* 31-37.

Rice, M. E. and Harris, G. T. (1997). Cross-validation and extension of the Violence Risk Appraisal Guide for child molesters and rapists. *Law and Human Behavior, 21*(2), 231-241.

Rice, M. E., Harris, G. T., and Quinsey, V. L. (1990). A follow-up of rapists assessed in a maximum-security psychiatric facility. *Journal of Interpersonal Violence, 5*(4), 435-448.

Righthand, S., Welch, C. M., Drach, K., Jacobs, J., Mosher, K., George, J., Kubik, E., and Roberson-Nay, R. (1998). *Child maltreatment risk, impact and intervention: Annotated bibliography.* Tyler, TX: Family Violence and Sexual Assault Institute.

Roche, D. N., Runtz, M. G., and Hunter, M. A. (1999). Adult attachment: A mediator between child sexual abuse and later psychological adjustment. *Journal of Interpersonal Violence, 14*(2), 184-207.

Rosenbaum, A. and O'Leary, D. (1981). Marital violence: characteristics of abusive couples. *Journal of Consulting and Clinical Psychology, 49*(1), 63-71.

Rosenstein, D. S. and Horowitz, H. A. (1996). Adolescent attachment and psychopathology. *Journal of Consulting and Clinical Psychology, 64*(2), 244-253.

Rotheram-Borus, M. J., Becker, J. V., Koopman, C., and Kaplan, M. (1991). AIDS knowledge and beliefs, and sexual behavior of sexually delinquent and nondelinquent (runaway) adolescents. *Journal of Adolescence, 14*(3), 229-244.

Rubin, K. H. and Lollis, S. P. (1988). Origins and consequences of social withdrawal. In J. Belsky and T. Nezworski (Eds.), *Clinical Implications of Attachment* (pp. 219-252). Hillsdale, NJ: Lawrence Erlbaum Associates.

Salekin, R. T., Rogers, R., and Sewell, K. W. (1996). A review and meta-analysis of the Psychopathy Checklist and Psychopathy Checklist-Revised: Predictive validity of dangerousness. *Clinical Psychology: Science and Practice, 3*(3), 203-215.

Saunders, B. E. (1997). Medical and mental health professionals as experts in legal cases. In P. Stern (Ed.), *Preparing and presenting expert testimony in child abuse litigation: A guide for expert witnesses and attorneys* (pp. 116-154). Thousand Oaks, CA: Sage Publications.

Saunders, B. E. and Williams, L. W. (Eds.) (1996). Treatment Outcome Research. *Child Maltreatment, 1*(4) (Special issue).

Saunders, D. G. (1995). Prediction of wife assault. In J. C. Campbell (Ed.), *Assessing dangerousness: Violence by sexual offenders, batterers, and child abusers* (pp. 68-95). Thousand Oaks, CA: Sage Publications.

Saunders, D. G. (1996). Feminist-cognitive-behavioral and process-psychodynamic treatments for men who batter: Interaction of abuser traits and treatment models. *Violence and Victims, 11*(4), 393-414.

Scalora, M. J. (1989, Summer). Assessing sex offenders' amenability to treatment: The need for professional modesty. *Expert Opinion: A newsletter of forensic mental health information for the Commonwealth of Massachusetts, 2*(4), 1, 4-6.

Schellenbach, C. J. (1998). Child maltreatment: A critical review of research on treatment for physically abusive parents. In P. K. Trickett and C. J. Schellenbach (Eds.), *Violence against children in the family and the community* (pp. 251-268). Washington, DC: American Psychological Association.

Schetky, D. H., Angell, R., Morrison, C. V., and Sack, W. H. (1979). Parents who fail: A study of 51 cases of termination of parental rights. *Journal of the American Academy of Child Psychiatry, 18*(2), 366-383.

Schram, D. D., Milloy, C. D., and Rowe, W. E. (1991). *Juvenile sex offenders: A follow-up study of reoffense behavior*. Olympia, WA: Washington State Institute for Public Policy.

Schuengel, C., Bakersman-Kranenburg, M. J., van IJzendoorn, M. H., and Blom, M. (1999). Unresolved loss and infant disorganization: Links to frightening maternal behavior. In J. Solomon and C. George (Eds.), *Attachment disorganization* (pp. 71-94). New York: The Guilford Press.

Schutz, B. M., Dixon, E. B., Lindenberger, J. C., and Ruther, N. J. (1989). *Solomon's sword: A practical guide to conducting child custody evaluations*. San Francisco, CA: Jossey-Bass Publishers.

Schwarz, E. D. and Perry, B. D. (1994). The post-traumatic response in children and adolescents. *Psychiatric Clinics of North America, 17*(2), 311-326.

Seagull, E. A. (1997). Family assessments. In M. E. Helfner, R. S. Kempe, and R. D. Krugman (Eds.), *The battered child,* Fifth edition (pp. 150-174). Chicago: University of Chicago Press.

Sedlack, A. J. and Broadhurst, D. D. (1996). *Third national incidence study of child abuse and neglect*. Washington, DC: United States Department of Health and Human Services.

Seidman, B. T., Marshall, W. L., Hudson, S. M., and Robertson, P. J. (1994). An examination of intimacy and loneliness in sex offenders. *Journal of Interpersonal Violence, 9*(4), 518-534.

Serin, R. C. (1996). Violent recidivism in criminal psychopaths. *Law and Human Behavior, 20*(2), 207-217.

Serin, R. C., Malcolm, P. B., Khanna, A., and Barbaree, H. E. (1994). Psychopathy and deviant sexual arousal in incarcerated sexual offenders. *Journal of Interpersonal Violence, 9*(1), 3-11.

Serin, R. C., Peters, R. D., and Barbaree, H. E. (1990). Predictors of psychopathy and release outcome in a criminal population. *Psychological Assessment: A Journal of Consulting and Clinical Psychology, 2*(4), 419-422.

Shipman, K. L., Rossman, B. B. R., and West, J. C. (1999). Co-occurrence of spousal violence and child abuse: Conceptual implications. *Child Maltreatment, 4*(2), 93-102.

Sipe, R., Jensen, E. L., and Everett, R. S. (1998). Adolescent sexual offenders grown up: Recidivism in young adulthood. *Criminal Justice and Behavior, 25*(1), 109-124.

Silvern, L., Karyl, J., Waelde, L., Hodges, W., Starek, J., Heidt, E., and Min, K. (1995). Retrospective reports of parental partner abuse: Relationships to depression, trauma symptoms and self-esteem among college students. *Journal of Family Violence, 10*(2), 177-202.

Simourd, D. J. (1997). The Criminal Sentiments Scale-Modified and Pride in Delinquency Scale: Psychometric properties and construct validity of two measures of criminal attitudes. *Criminal Justice and Behavior, 24,* 52-70.

Smith, D. T. (1991). Parent-child interaction play assessment. In G. E. Shafer, K. Gitlin, and A. Sandgrund (Eds.), *Play diagnosis and assessment* (pp. 463-492). New York: Wiley and Sons.

Smith, W. R. and Monastersky, C. (1986). Assessing juvenile sexual offenders' risk for reoffending. *Criminal Justice and Behavior, 13*(2), 115-140.

Solomon, C. R. and Serres, F. (1999). Effects of parental verbal aggression on children's self-esteem and school marks. *Child Abuse and Neglect, 23*(4), 339-351.

Solomon, J. and George, C. (1999). The measurement of attachment security in infancy and childhood. In J. Cassidy and P. R. Shaver (Eds.), *Handbook of attachment: Theory, research, and clinical applications* (pp. 287-316). New York: The Guilford Press.

Stamm, H. (Ed.) (1996). *Measurement of stress, trauma, and adaptation.* Lutherville, MD: The Sidran Press.

State Forensic Service (1995). *Sex offender assessment program policies and procedures.* Augusta, ME: Author.

Steadman, H. J., Mulvey, E. P., Monahan, J., Robbins, P. C., Applebaum, P. S., Grisso, T., Roth, L. H., and Silver, E. (1998). Violence by people discharged from acute psychiatric inpatient facilities and by others in the same neighborhoods. *Archives of General Psychiatry, 55*(5), 393-401.

Steadman, H. J., Silver, E., Monahan, J., Appelbaum, P. S., Robbins, P. C., Mulvey, E. P., Grisso, T., Roth, L. H., and Banks, S. (2000). A classification tree approach to the development of actuarial violence risk assessment tools. *Law and Human Behavior, 24*(1), 83-100.

Stermac, L. and Sheridan, L. (1993). The developmentally disabled adolescent sex offender. In H. E. Barbaree, W. L. Marshall, and S. M. Hudson (Eds.), *The juvenile sex offender* (pp. 235-242). New York: The Guilford Press.

Stern, P. (1997). *Preparing and presenting expert testimony in child abuse litigation: A guide for expert witnesses and attorneys.* Thousand Oaks, CA: Sage Publications.

Sternberg, K. J., Lamb, M. E., Greenbaum, C., Cicchetti, D., Dawud, S., Cortes, R. M., Krispin, O., and Lorey, F. (1993). Effects of domestic violence on children's behavior problems and depression. *Developmental Psychology, 29*(1), 44-52.

Sudermann, M. and Jaffe, P. (1997). Children and youth who witness violence: New directions in intervention and prevention. In D. Wolfe, R. J. McMahon, and R. DeV. Peters (Eds.), *Child abuse: New directions in prevention and treatment across the lifespan* (pp. 55-78). Thousand Oaks, CA: Sage Publications.

Sullivan, C. M., Juras, J., Bybee, D., Nguyen, H., and Allen, A. (2000). How children's adjustment is affected by their relationships to their mothers' abusers. *Journal of Interpersonal Violence, 15*(6), 587-602.

Swanson, J. W. (1994). Mental disorder, substance abuse, and community violence: An epidemiological approach. In J. Monahan and H. J. Steadman (Eds.), *Violence and mental disorder: Developments in risk assessment* (pp. 101-136). Chicago: University of Chicago Press.

Swanson, M. C. J., Bland, R. C., and Newman, S. C. (1994). Antisocial Personality Disorders. *Acta Psychiatrica Sandanavica, 89*(376, Suppl.), 63-70.

Thorpe, G. L., Righthand, S., and Kubik, E. K. (2001). Dimensions of burnout in professionals working with sex offenders. *Sexual Abuse: A Journal of Research and Treatment, 13*(3).

Toth, S. L., Manly, J. T., and Cicchetti, D. (1992). Child maltreatment and vulnerability to depression. *Development and Psychopathology, 4*(1), 97-112.

Tyler, K. A., Hoyt, D. R., and Whitbeck, L. B. (2000). The effects of early sexual abuse on later sexual victimization among female homeless and runaway adolescents. *Journal of Interpersonal Violence, 15*(3), 235-250.

Tymchuk, A. J. (1992). Predicting adequacy of parenting by people with mental retardation. *Child Abuse and Neglect, 16*(2), 165-178.

Tymchuk, A. J. and Feldman, M. A. (1991). Parents with mental retardation and their children: Review of research relevant to professional practice. *Canadian Psychology, 32*(3), 486-494.

Tymchuk, A. J., Hamada, D., Andron, L., and Anderson, S. (1990). Home safety training with mothers who are mentally retarded. *Education and Training in Mental Retardation, 25*(2), 142-149.

U.S. Department of Health and Human Services Administration for Children and Families (1995). *A nation's shame: Fatal child abuse and neglect in the United States: A report of the U.S. Advisory Board on Child Abuse and Neglect.* Washington, DC: U.S. Government Printing Office.

van IJzendoorn, M. H. and Bakermans-Kranenburg, M. J. (1996). Attachment representations in mothers, fathers, adolescents, and clinical groups: A meta-analytic search for normative data. *Journal of Consulting and Clinical Psychology,* *64*(1), 8-21.

Visard, E., Monck, E., and Misch, P. (1995). Child and adolescent sex abuse perpetrators: A review of the research literature. *Journal of Child Psychology and Psychiatry, 36*(5), 731-756.

Vissing, Y. M., Straus, M. A., Gelles, R., and Harrop, J. W. (1991). Verbal aggression by parents and psychosocial problems of children. *Child Abuse and Neglect, 15*(3), 223-238.

Volavka, J. (1995). *Neurobiology of violence.* Washington, DC: American Psychiatric Press, Inc.

Wagner, W. G., Aucoin, R., and Johnson, J. T. (1993). Psychologists' attitudes concerning child sexual abuse: The impact of sex of perpetrator, sex of victim, age of victim, and victim response. *Journal of Child Sexual Abuse, 2*(2), 61-74.

Ward, T. and Hudson, S. (1998). A model of the relapse process in sexual offenders. *Journal of Interpersonal Violence, 13*(6), 700-725.

Warner, J. D., Malinosky-Rummell, R., Ellis, J. T., and Hansen, D. J. (1990). An examination of demographic and treatment variables associated with session attendance of maltreating families. Paper presented at the annual conference of the Association for the Advancement of Behavior Therapy, San Francisco, November.

Waterman, C. K. and Foss-Goodman, D. (1984). Child molesting: Variables relating to attribution of fault to victims, offenders, and nonparticipating parents. The *Journal of Sex Research, 20*(4), 329-349.

Webster, C. D., Douglas, K. S., Eaves, D., and Hart, S. D. (1997a). *The HCR-20: Assessment risk for violence, Version 2.* Burnaby, British Columbia: Mental Health, Law, and Policy Institute, Simon Fraser University and Forensic Psychiatric Services Commission of British Columbia.

Webster, C. D., Douglas, K. S., Eaves, D., and Hart, S. D. (1997b). Assessing risk of violence to others. In C. D. Webster and M. A. Jackson (Eds.), *Impulsivity: Theory, assessment, and treatment* (pp. 251-277). New York: The Guilford Press.

Webster, C. D., Eaves, D., Douglas, K., and Wintrup, A. (1995). *The HCR-20 scheme: The assessment of dangerousness and risk.* Vancouver, Canada: Simon Fraser University and Forensic Psychiatric Services Commission of British Columbia.

Webster, C. D., Harris, G. T., Rice, M. E., Cormier, C., and Quinsey, V. L. (1994). *The violence prediction scheme: Assessing dangerousness in high risk men.* Toronto: University of Toronto.

Weeks, R. and Widom, C. S. (1998). Self-reports of early childhood victimization among incarcerated adult felons. *Journal of Interpersonal Violence, 13*(3), 346-361.

Weinrott, M. (1996). *Juvenile sexual aggression: A critical review.* Boulder, CO: University of Colorado, Institute for Behavioral Sciences, Center for the Study and Prevention of Violence.

Wekerle, C. and Wolfe, D. A. (1993). Prevention of child physical abuse and neglect: Promising new directions. *Clinical Psychology Review, 13*(6), 501-540.

Werner, E. E. (1989). High-risk children in young adulthood: a longitudinal study from birth to 32 years. *American Journal of Orthopsychiatry, 59*(1), 72-81.

White, R. and Gondolf, E. (2000). Implications of personality profiles for batterer treatment: Support for the gender-based, cognitive-behavioral approach. *Journal of Interpersonal Violence, 15*(5), 467-488.

Widom, C. S. (1989). Does violence beget violence? A critical examination of the literature. *Psychological Bulletin, 106*(1), 3-28.

Widom, C. S. (1999). Posttraumatic stress disorder in abused and neglected children grown up. *American Journal of Psychiatry, 156*(8), 1223-1229.

Wind, T. W. and Silvern, L. (1992). Type and extent of child abuse as predictors of adult functioning. *Journal of Family Violence, 7*(4), 261-281.

Wind, T. W. and Silvern, L. (1994). Parenting and the effects of abuse. *Child Abuse and Neglect, 18*(5), 439-453.

Wolfe, D. A. (1985). Child-abusive parents: An empirical review and analysis. *Psychological Bulletin, 97*(3), 462-482.

Wolfe, D. A. (1987). Child abuse: Implications for child development and psychopathology. *Developmental Clinical Psychology and Psychiatry, 10* (Special issue).

Wolfe, D. A. (1991). *Preventing physical and emotional abuse of children.* New York: The Guilford Press.

Wolfe, D. A. (1994). The role of intervention and treatment services in the prevention of child abuse and neglect. In G. B. Melton and F. D. Barry (Eds.), *Protecting children from abuse and neglect: Foundations for a new national strategy* (pp. 224-303). New York: The Guilford Press.

Wolfe, D. A., Aragona, J., Kaufman, K., and Sandler, J. (1980). The importance of adjudication in the treatment of child abusers: Some preliminary findings. *Child Abuse and Neglect, 4,* 127-135.

Wolfe, D. A. and Wekerle, C. (1993). Treatment strategies for child physical abuse and neglect: A critical progress report. *Clinical Psychology Review, 13*(6), 473-500.

Wolfner, G. D., and Gelles, R. J. (1993). A profile of violence toward children: A national study. *Child Abuse and Neglect, 17*(2), 197-212.

Worling, J. R. and Curwen, T. (2000). Adolescent sexual offender recidivism: Success of specialized treatment and implications for risk prediction. *Child Abuse and Neglect, 24*(7), 965-982.

Worling, J. R. and Curwen, T. (2001). Estimate of risk of adolescent sexual offense recidivism (Version 2.0: The "ERASOR"). In M.C. Calder, *Juveniles and children who sexually abuse: Frameworks for assessment* (pp. 372-397). Lyme Regis, Dorset, UK: Russell House Publishing.

Yoast, R. A. and McIntyre, K. (1991). *Alcohol, other drug abuse and child abuse and neglect.* Madison, WI: Wisconsin Clearing House, University of Wisconsin-Madison.

Youngblade, L. M. and Belsky, J. (1989). Child maltreatment, infant-parent attachment security, and dysfunctional peer relationships in toddlerhood. *Topics in Early Childhood Special Education, 9*(2), 1-15.

Zuravin, S., McMillen, C., DePanfilis, D., and Risley-Curtiss, C. (1996). The intergenerational cycle of child maltreatment: Continuity versus discontinuity. *Journal of Interpersonal Violence, 11*(3), 315-335.

Zuravin, S. J. and Starr, R. H. Jr. (1991). Psychosocial characteristics of mothers of physically abused and neglected children: Do they differ by race? In R. L. Hampton (Ed.), *Black family violence: Current research and theory* (37-71). Lexington, MA: Lexington Books.

Index

THE HAWORTH MALTREATMENT AND TRAUMA PRESS®
Robert A. Geffner, PhD
Senior Editor

CHILD MALTREATMENT RISK ASSESSMENTS: AN EVALUATION GUIDE by Sue Righthand, Bruce Kerr, and Kerry Drach. (2003). "This book is essential reading for clinicians and forensic examiners who see cases involving issues related to child maltreatment. The authors have compiled an impressive critical survey of the relevant research on child maltreatment. Their material is well organized into sections on definitions, impact, risk assessment, and risk management. This book represents a giant step toward promoting evidence-based evaluations, treatment, and testimony." *Diane H. Schetky, MD, Professor of Psychiatry, University of Vermont College of Medicine*

SIMPLE AND COMPLEX POST-TRAUMATIC STRESS DISORDER: STRATEGIES FOR COMPREHENSIVE TREATMENT IN CLINICAL PRACTICE edited by Mary Beth Williams and John F. Sommer Jr. (2002). "A welcome addition to the literature on treating survivors of traumatic events, this volume possesses all the ingredients necessary for even the experienced clinician to master the management of patients with PTSD." *Terence M. Keane, PhD, Chief, Psychology Service, VA Boston Healthcare System; Professor and Vice Chair of Research in Psychiatry, Boston University School of Medicine*

FOR LOVE OF COUNTRY: CONFRONTING RAPE AND SEXUAL HARASSMENT IN THE U.S. MILITARY by T. S. Nelson. (2002). "Nelson brings an important message—that the absence of current media attention doesn't mean the problem has gone away; that only decisive action by military leadership at all levels can break the cycle of repeated traumatization; and that the failure to do so is, as Nelson puts it, a 'power failure'—a refusal to exert positive leadership at all levels to stop violent individuals from using the worst power imaginable." *Chris Lombardi, Correspondent, Women's E-News, New York City*

THE INSIDERS: A MAN'S RECOVERY FROM TRAUMATIC CHILDHOOD ABUSE by Robert Blackburn Knight. (2002). "An important book. . . . Fills a gap in the literature about healing from childhood sexual abuse by allowing us to hear, in undiluted terms, about one man's history and journey of recovery." *Amy Pine, MA, LMFT, psychotherapist and co-founder, Survivors Healing Center, Santa Cruz, California*

WE ARE NOT ALONE: A GUIDEBOOK FOR HELPING PROFESSIONALS AND PARENTS SUPPORTING ADOLESCENT VICTIMS OF SEXUAL ABUSE by Jade Christine Angelica. (2002). "Encourages victims and their families to participate in the system in an effort to heal from their victimization, seek justice, and hold offenders accountable for their crimes. An exceedingly vital training tool." *Janet Fine, MS, Director, Victim Witness Assistance Program and Children's Advocacy Center, Suffolk County District Attorney's Office, Boston*

WE ARE NOT ALONE: A TEENAGE GIRL'S PERSONAL ACCOUNT OF INCEST FROM DISCLOSURE THROUGH PROSECUTION AND TREATMENT by Jade Christine Angelica. (2002). "A valuable resource for teens who have been sexually abused and their parents. With compassion and eloquent prose, Angelica walks people through the criminal justice system—from disclosure to final outcome." *Kathleen Kendall-Tackett, PhD, Research Associate, Family Research Laboratory, University of New Hampshire, Durham*

WE ARE NOT ALONE: A TEENAGE BOY'S PERSONAL ACCOUNT OF CHILD SEXUAL ABUSE FROM DISCLOSURE THROUGH PROSECUTION AND TREATMENT by Jade Christine Angelica. (2002). "Inspires us to work harder to meet kids' needs, answer their questions, calm their fears, and protect them from their abusers and the system, which is often not designed to respond to them in a language they understand." *Kevin L. Ryle, JD, Assistant District Attorney, Middlesex, Massachusetts*

GROWING FREE: A MANUAL FOR SURVIVORS OF DOMESTIC VIOLENCE by Wendy Susan Deaton and Michael Hertica. (2001). "This is a necessary book for anyone who is scared and starting to think about what it would take to 'grow free.' . . . Very helpful for friends and relatives of a person in a domestic violence situation. I recommend it highly." *Colleen Friend, LCSW, Field Work Consultant, UCLA Department of Social Welfare, School of Public Policy & Social Research*

A THERAPIST'S GUIDE TO GROWING FREE: A MANUAL FOR SURVIVOR'S OF DOMESTIC VIOLENCE by Wendy Susan Deaton and Michael Hertica. (2001). "An excellent synopsis of the theories and research behind the manual." *Beatrice Crofts Yorker, RN, JD, Professor of Nursing, Georgia State University, Decatur*

PATTERNS OF CHILD ABUSE: HOW DYSFUNCTIONAL TRANSACTIONS ARE REPLICATED IN INDIVIDUALS, FAMILIES, AND THE CHILD WELFARE SYSTEM by Michael Karson. (2001). "No one interested in what may well be the major public health epidemic of our time in terms of its long-term consequences for our society can afford to pass up the opportunity to read this enlightening work." *Howard Wolowitz, PhD, Professor Emeritus, Psychology Department, University of Michigan, Ann Arbor*

IDENTIFYING CHILD MOLESTERS: PREVENTING CHILD SEXUAL ABUSE BY RECOGNIZING THE PATTERNS OF THE OFFENDERS by Carla van Dam. (2000). "The definitive work on the subject. . . . Provides parents and others with the tools to recognize when and how to intervene." *Roger W. Wolfe, MA, Co-Director, N. W. Treatment Associates, Seattle, Washington*

POLITICAL VIOLENCE AND THE PALESTINIAN FAMILY: IMPLICATIONS FOR MENTAL HEALTH AND WELL-BEING by Vivian Khamis. (2000). "A valuable book . . . a pioneering work that fills a glaring gap in the study of Palestinian society." *Elia Zureik, Professor of Sociology, Queens University, Kingston, Ontario, Canada*

STOPPING THE VIOLENCE: A GROUP MODEL TO CHANGE MEN'S ABUSIVE ATTITUDES AND BEHAVIORS by David J. Decker. (1999). "A concise and thorough manual to assist clinicians in learning the causes and dynamics of domestic violence." *Joanne Kittel, MSW, LICSW, Yachats, Oregon*

STOPPING THE VIOLENCE: A GROUP MODEL TO CHANGE MEN'S ABUSIVE ATTITUDES AND BEHAVIORS, THE CLIENT WORKBOOK by David J. Decker. (1999).

BREAKING THE SILENCE: GROUP THERAPY FOR CHILDHOOD SEXUAL ABUSE, A PRACTITIONER'S MANUAL by Judith A. Margolin. (1999). "This book is an extremely valuable and well-written resource for all therapists working with adult survivors of child sexual abuse." *Esther Deblinger, PhD, Associate Professor of Clinical Psychiatry, University of Medicine and Dentistry of New Jersey School of Osteopathic Medicine*

"I NEVER TOLD ANYONE THIS BEFORE": MANAGING THE INITIAL DISCLOSURE OF SEXUAL ABUSE RE-COLLECTIONS by Janice A. Gasker. (1999). "Discusses the elements needed to create a safe, therapeutic environment and offers the practitioner a number of useful strategies for responding appropriately to client disclosure." *Roberta G. Sands, PhD, Associate Professor, University of Pennsylvania School of Social Work*

FROM SURVIVING TO THRIVING: A THERAPIST'S GUIDE TO STAGE II RECOVERY FOR SURVIVORS OF CHILDHOOD ABUSE by Mary Bratton. (1999). "A must read for all, including survivors. Bratton takes a lifelong debilitating disorder and unravels its intricacies in concise, succinct, and understandable language." *Phillip A. Whitner, PhD, Sr. Staff Counselor, University Counseling Center, The University of Toledo, Ohio*

SIBLING ABUSE TRAUMA: ASSESSMENT AND INTERVENTION STRATEGIES FOR CHILDREN, FAMILIES, AND ADULTS by John V. Caffaro and Allison Conn-Caffaro. (1998). "One area that has almost consistently been ignored in the research and writing on child maltreatment is the area of sibling abuse. This book is a welcome and required addition to the developing literature on abuse." *Judith L. Alpert, PhD, Professor of Applied Psychology, New York University*

BEARING WITNESS: VIOLENCE AND COLLECTIVE RESPONSIBILITY by Sandra L. Bloom and Michael Reichert. (1998). "A totally convincing argument. . . . Demands careful study by all elected representatives, the clergy, the mental health and medical professions, representatives of the media, and all those unwittingly involved in this repressive perpetuation and catastrophic global problem." *Harold I. Eist, MD, Past President, American Psychiatric Association*

TREATING CHILDREN WITH SEXUALLY ABUSIVE BEHAVIOR PROBLEMS: GUIDELINES FOR CHILD AND PARENT INTERVENTION by Jan Ellen Burton, Lucinda A. Rasmussen, Julie Bradshaw, Barbara J. Christopherson, and Steven C. Huke. (1998). "An extremely readable book that is well-documented and a mine of valuable 'hands on' information. . . . This is a book that all those who work with sexually abusive children or want to work with them must read." *Sharon K. Araji, PhD, Professor of Sociology, University of Alaska, Anchorage*

THE LEARNING ABOUT MYSELF (LAMS) PROGRAM FOR AT-RISK PARENTS: LEARNING FROM THE PAST—CHANGING THE FUTURE by Verna Rickard. (1998). "This program should be a part of the resource materials of every mental health professional trusted with the responsibility of working with 'at-risk' parents." *Terry King, PhD, Clinical Psychologist, Federal Bureau of Prisons, Catlettsburg, Kentucky*

THE LEARNING ABOUT MYSELF (LAMS) PROGRAM FOR AT-RISK PARENTS: HANDBOOK FOR GROUP PARTICIPANTS by Verna Rickard. (1998). "Not only is the LAMS program designed to be educational and build skills for future use, it is also fun!" *Martha Morrison Dore, PhD, Associate Professor of Social Work, Columbia University, New York, New York*

BRIDGING WORLDS: UNDERSTANDING AND FACILITATING ADOLESCENT RECOVERY FROM THE TRAUMA OF ABUSE by Joycee Kennedy and Carol McCarthy. (1998). "An extraordinary survey of the history of child neglect and abuse in America. . . . A wonderful teaching tool at the university level, but should be required reading in high schools as well." *Florabel Kinsler, PhD, BCD, LCSW, Licensed Clinical Social Worker, Los Angeles, California*

CEDAR HOUSE: A MODEL CHILD ABUSE TREATMENT PROGRAM by Bobbi Kendig with Clara Lowry. (1998). "Kendig and Lowry truly . . . realize the saying that we are our brothers' keepers. Their spirit permeates this volume, and that spirit of caring is what always makes the difference for people in painful situations." *Hershel K. Swinger, PhD, Clinical Director, Children's Institute International, Los Angeles, California*

SEXUAL, PHYSICAL, AND EMOTIONAL ABUSE IN OUT-OF-HOME CARE: PREVENTION SKILLS FOR AT-RISK CHILDREN by Toni Cavanagh Johnson and Associates. (1997). "Professionals who make dispositional decisions or who are related to out-of-home care for children could benefit from reading and following the curriculum of this book with children in placements." *Issues in Child Abuse Accusations*